WHEN FOOD
BITES BACK

Taking Control of Autoimmune Disease

Elroy Vojdani, MD, IFMCP

Mention of specific companies, organizations, or authorities in this book does not imply endorsement by the author or publisher. Information in this book was accurate at the time researched. The author received no incentives or compensation to promote the item recommendations in the book. Names in case studies have been changed to protect the parties.
Library of Congress Cataloging-in-Publication Data is on file with the publisher

When Food Bites Back / Elroy Vojdani, MD, IFMCP
ISBN: 978-0-578-33185-0
1. Health 2. Diet 3. Autoimmunity 4. Biology

Cover design: Spotlight Group Agency

To my father, Aristo Vojdani, PhD,
the father of functional immunology—
a pioneer from day one and fearless the entire way.

TABLE OF CONTENTS

FOREWORD

Fundamental to the survival and ultimate success of the human species is our ability to rapidly distinguish between friend and foe. And while we, like other species, benefit from our ability to aid and cooperate with our conspecifics, we humans clearly differentiate ourselves from other species in terms of the degree by which we can harm them. So, much is riding on the outcome of the friend or foe dichotomy.

Similarly, the myriad components of our immune systems make rapid friend or foe decisions countless times each day as we interact with our environment. Our immune systems are vigilantly surveying our environment moment to moment through a variety of interfaces, including lung tissue, which processes airborne chemical and cellular information through lung-related immune cells.

Similarly to how we respond to airborne substances, our bodies can discern whether chemical components of the foods we consume are beneficial or threatening. This remarkable and virtually instantaneous process has been highly refined through millions of years of evolution.

We eat foods to harvest the nutrients they contain, including the macronutrients fat, protein, and carbohydrates, as well as various micronutrients, including vitamins and minerals. While we know food provides building blocks and energy sources for our bodies, we've now gained an understanding of the role of food as a deeply instructive source of information. In other words, food doesn't just serve as raw materials and fuel; rather, it relays up-to-date information about our environment, modifying the functionality of our immune systems, and even nuancing the expression of our DNA—our life code—so as to harmonize our most fundamental life processes with the environment in which we live.

In modern Western medicine, embracing the notion of a profound interaction between food and immune function threatens the bedrock reductionist mentality that so pervades both the practice of medicine as well as its antecedent educational process. The notion of common ground between the gastroenterologist and immunologist still rings challenging. And yet, as you will soon learn, not only do unique characteristics of specific foods dramatically affect immune regulation but, more importantly, the relationship between food and the immune system is fully bidirectional, as a host of extrinsic influences on the immune system play upon how our food choices are embraced.

The pages that follow reveal how a vast number of common experiences that characterize our modern world, from air fresheners to food additives, tinker with the immune system's ability to make the friend or foe decision. This then leads to both the lack of a meaningful immune response to potentially threatening confrontations as well as misguided, overactive, and inappropriate responses against our very own tissue—the definition of autoimmunity.

What Dr. Elroy Vojdani has gifted us in this book is not only a fount of information allowing us to get our arms around this seemingly complex science but, most importantly, a welcomed road map that allows each of us the ability to re-establish balance in our immune functionality. The value of this gift cannot be overstated, as immune dysregulation represents the cornerstone of the most pervasive health challenges of our modern world.

Yes, "food is medicine." But it is only medicine when it is fully appreciated for all it represents, including how it is interpreted by the immune system. And this so deeply highlights the value of looking upon this remarkable human body as a fully integrated whole.

David Perlmutter, MD
Naples, Florida
May 2021

Introduction

LET THE HEALING JOURNEY BEGIN

*The doctor of the future will give no medicine but will
instruct his patient in the care of the human frame, in diet,
and in the cause and prevention of disease.*

– Thomas Edison

The path to this book began with my paternal grandmother's plight with rheumatoid arthritis. She began showing symptoms two years after developing an oral infection from shoddy dentistry. She was only forty-five, and her symptoms gradually and painfully worsened with each passing year until she became so disabled she needed a total knee replacement.

Witnessing his mother's steady decline motivated my father to become an immunologist. He believed that if he could discover the root cause of her condition, he could help her reverse it. He accompanied her to the hospital and orthopedic and rheumatologic clinics, carefully questioning her surgeons and physicians. To his dismay, her doctors either professed not to know the cause of her condition or simply attributed it to genetics. Since none of my grandmother's siblings nor any of her ten children had the disease, my father rejected this diagnosis. He suspected it had something to do with her past dental history, but no other doctor agreed.

While working on his PhD, my father heard a lecture on the connection between streptococcal infection, rheumatic fever, and autoimmune disease. It was an "Aha!" moment that inspired his own theory on the cause-and-effect relationship between infection and rheumatoid arthritis. He collected blood samples from his mother and three healthy subjects to perform antibody analyses against a variety of pathogens (bacteria, viruses, or other microorganisms that can cause disease). The specimens from the three healthy controls registered antibodies in the normal range. However, in my grandmother's blood sample, my father found increased antibodies for *Staphylococcus* (the bacterium that causes staph infections), *Klebsiella* (a gut bacterium that can lead to urinary tract infections), *Yersinia* (a pathogen found in raw or undercooked pork), *E. coli* (a gut bacterium commonly found in contaminated foods), *Streptococcus mutans* (the leading cause of dental caries), and *Porphyromonas* (another oral pathogen). The results convinced my father that chronic infection played a role in the development of my grandmother's autoimmune disease. He also noticed that certain foods—milk, cereals, egg, codfish, red meat, and nightshade vegetables—exacerbated her symptoms. These revelations began my father's lifelong mission to demystify the root causes behind autoimmunity.

Today, my father, Dr. Aristo Vojdani, is widely recognized in the medical science field as "the father of functional immunology." Over the years, he played an active role in developing highly advanced testing for food reactivity and led the way to incredible breakthroughs in the study of immunology. His ongoing research continues to focus on the role of environmental triggers in complex diseases, and he holds fifteen U.S. patents for laboratory assessments of immune disorders associated with the gut and brain. He is also the founder of Immunosciences Lab Inc. in Los Angeles, California, and serves as chief scientific advisor at Cyrex Laboratories in Phoenix, Arizona.

When I was a child, our family dinner conversations typically started with light banter and inevitably progressed into the heady realm of the latest scientific and medical trends. I absorbed every word my father said (even those that went over my head at the time) with great interest and passion. As a teenager, I assisted my father in his laboratory, where I learned how to conduct and read diagnostic tests. Later, I joined him at medical conferences and watched in awe as industry giants listened and learned from him. My father's good work inspired me to walk in his footsteps.

When I entered the hectic grind of medical school, I gained weight and experienced mental fatigue and monthly sinus infections. When my father ran a simple blood test on me, it revealed that I had significant immune reactivity to both dairy and gluten. Sure enough, my symptoms abated as soon as I removed the offending foods from my diet. After reclaiming my health, I went on to become an interventional radiologist, diagnosing and treating complex, late-stage cancers and other debilitating diseases. Though I witnessed truly incredible developments that saved people's lives, I kept coming back to my first love, immunology—but more specifically, functional immunology.

When practiced properly, functional medicine can be life-changing. Rather than looking at the body as individual parts and writing prescriptions to mask symptoms, functional medicine focuses on the body as a whole system. What's more, it seeks to identify the root causes driving disease through cutting-edge science, state-of-the-art medical testing, and keen observation. This powerful approach includes a preventive aspect. When armed with the right information, you can sidestep disease from taking hold in the first place—even if you're genetically predisposed to certain illnesses.

Maybe you're also experiencing symptoms of autoimmune dysfunction, such as fatigue, headaches, and brain fog, or skin rashes, stomach upset, and muscle aches. Perhaps you've run from doctor to doctor in search of answers, only to leave with a handful of prescriptions and blood tests results that fall within the so-called "normal" range. It's likely you've been made to believe your aches and pains are all in your head. Or maybe you've been diagnosed with one of the more than 100 known autoimmune diseases—lupus, thyroiditis, or irritable bowel syndrome, to name a few—and you sense there's a better way to manage your condition than with conventional medicine alone. If so, you've come to the right place.

In my practice at Regenera Medical in Los Angeles, California, I receive daily confirmation that functional medicine is without question the future of health care. Patients come to me at their wits' end trying to find the cause of their untreated or misdiagnosed chronic medical condition(s), including migraines, brain fog, psoriasis, thyroid imbalance, unexplained weight gain, digestive issues, and exhaustion. My medical training, along with my background in radiology and deep understanding of how blood tests are created and conducted, allows me to accurately diagnose patients and customize an effective treatment plan. Over and over again, the answer almost always comes down to the foods and beverages we are putting into our bodies.

Autoimmunity is a complex beast, with many variables such as genetics, stress, insulin resistance, and poor sleep habits. Still, the food we consume is by far the single greatest contributing factor, and more than 70 percent of autoimmune disorders can be traced back to consuming the wrong foods. Even if diabetes runs in your family and you are genetically predisposed, that doesn't necessarily mean you will develop the disease. An environmental trigger must turn that gene on, and more often than not, that trigger is a combination of foods that turn the immune system against the body it is designed to protect.

This book focuses on food-related autoimmunity. It is also a labor of love to motivate a favorable lifestyle shift that significantly benefits both mind and body. The average patient with autoimmune disease sees six doctors over the course of five years before receiving a correct diagnosis. Many compare the process to traveling on a road where you have no control, but this book seeks to address and correct that. Within these pages, you'll learn how to go beyond blindly following doctors' orders. You'll discover how to find a qualified practitioner and how to work in partnership with them. You may also learn discouraging information, such as the dangers of sugar, salt, gluten, dairy, lectins, and more. But once you experience positive outcomes like clear thinking and boundless energy again, I promise you won't miss the french fries, gluten-filled pizza dough, or mucus-causing ice cream as much as you thought you might. Even if you're already eating clean, you'll discover how to fine-tune your diet for optimal health.

DETECT, REMOVE, AND REPAIR

While I was writing this book in early 2021, the COVID-19 pandemic was in full swing. Many of us have read about the Spanish flu of 1918; yes, humans bounced back, and we will again. But what we've seen with COVID-19 underscores the importance of protecting our bodies from underlying conditions that can literally make the difference between life and death.

As the pandemic unfolded before our eyes, many of us in the United States realized our country had reached a dangerous tipping point. Never before in our lifetimes has it been so obvious that each of us needs to be proactive in nurturing our immune systems. The evidence clearly shows that people who do not suffer from inflammatory, cardiovascular, or immunological diseases fare much better with COVID-19 infection than those who do.

Worldwide, about 10 percent of the population exhibits symptoms of autoimmunity. In the United States, research reveals that one in six people (countless more if you consider those who have not been diagnosed) are afflicted—and that number continues to grow.

Throughout human existence, our bodies and DNA have adapted to the food we eat, creating tolerances and enabling our species to thrive. The structure of *Homo sapiens* has progressed over the course of 300,000 years, but in the last century, our bodies have been forced to adapt to drastic environmental shifts in what is a speck of time, relatively. Sadly, our species is not able to adapt at such a rapid pace, especially in the face of new, hybridized, and heavily processed foods.

Over the past decade, cases of chronic illness, obesity, diabetes, Alzheimer's, inflammatory bowel syndrome, and other diseases categorized as "immunocompromised" have risen sharply. According to the National Institutes of Health (NIH), 25.3 million Americans currently live with an autoimmune disorder. The agency only accounts for twenty-three disorders in their statistics, so when you take into account the other sixty-plus autoimmune diseases and those that are undiagnosed or misdiagnosed, the actual number is closer to 50 million.

Obesity is an inflammatory disease with an upregulated and imbalanced immune system, as are cardiovascular diseases and autoimmune disorders. The good news is functional medicine knows more about autoimmunity than ever before. We can intervene and control it before irreversible damage sets in. The answer lies in the three pillars for re-establishing gut health:

- Detect the problem
- Remove the triggers
- Repair the barrier

Autoimmune disease can be silent or relatively silent for ten or fifteen years before symptoms appear, but the earlier you act, the better off you're going to be. If you're already living with a diagnosed condition, understanding the origins of autoimmunity and the inner workings of your immune system will be key to liberating yourself. It may seem like a huge undertaking, but with the right choices, the human body is resilient and can heal. What's key is arming yourself with the knowledge and power to take action. Here's a quick look at some of the main themes we'll be covering.

This book is organized into four sections: Autoimmunity 101, Detect the Problem, Remove the Triggers, and Repair the Barrier. We'll begin the healing journey with a self-assessment to determine your risk for autoimmunity. This will include evaluating family history, diet, stress levels, sleep hygiene, bowel habits, symptoms, and more. Please fill out the survey before you read on and then revisit your responses in ninety days to evaluate your progress.

Autoimmunity 101: In Chapter 1, "The Silent Epidemic," we'll explore what autoimmunity is and how it develops. In Chapter 2, "The Immune System," we'll tour the complex army of cells, chemicals, and organs charged with protecting your body from invading toxins and pathogens. In Chapter 3, "The Digestive System," we'll look at digestive health and elaborate on leaky gut, the primary driver behind autoimmunity.

Detect the Problem: In Chapter 4, "Be Your Own Medical Detective," you'll learn about the power of predictive testing, as well as the latest diagnostic tests available for identifying leaky gut and food-related autoimmunity. We'll also touch on the pros and cons of elimination diets and how to follow them properly. In Chapters 5 through 8, we'll look at some of the more common autoimmune disorders affecting the gastrointestinal tract, brain and nervous system, thyroid, joints, and skin, and meet some of my patients who put their symptoms into remission, or, in some cases, completely eliminated them. I hope their successes serve as inspiration for your own journey as you discover how to take control of your health.

Remove the Triggers: In Chapter 10, "Smoothing the Transition," you'll discover tips and insights on how to navigate the healing transition during the elimination phase. In Chapters 11 through 14, we'll examine some of the most common food triggers—wheat, dairy, eggs, legumes, nightshade vegetables, and additives like sugar, salt, gums, food coloring, meat and food glue, and more—and learn how they contribute to inflammation and autoimmunity.

Repair the Barrier: In Chapter 15, "Eating to Thrive," you'll read about foods that act as medicine for your body. And finally, in Chapter 16's "Gut-Healing Supplements," we'll look at the vitamins, minerals, and probiotics that promote vibrant, glowing health.

NOTES

NOTES

SELF-ASSESSMENT SURVEY

Whenever I meet with a new patient, I always begin by evaluating their vulnerabilities for autoimmune disease. We look at symptoms, genetics, lifestyle, stress levels, relationships, and their home environment. Here, I've modified my patient questionnaire so you can go through this process on your own. For each question, answer Yes for often, Sometimes for somewhat, and No for never or rarely. Pay attention to sections containing a concentration of Y answers. This is a good place to take stock of your diet and lifestyle habits, set goals for improvement, and help you identify which areas to place the most emphasis on during your healing journey. Be sure revisit this survey in ninety days to monitor your progress.

SYMPTOMS	DATE:	DATE (90+ DAYS):

GASTROINTESTINAL

CHECK ALL THAT APPLY

- Heartburn ☐
- Bad breath ☐
- Skin rashes ☐
- Hemorrhoids ☐
- Distended stomach ☐
- Puffy eyes ☐
- Dark circles under eyes ☐
- Frequent fever or chills ☐
- Abdominal pain or cramping ☐
- Burning in stomach if haven't eaten for a while ☐
- Nausea or the feeling that you may vomit ☐
- Sense of being full after eating a small amount ☐
- Frequent gas, flatulence, or burping ☐
- Bloating, headaches, stomach pain, or skin rash after eating a particular food ☐
- Hard stools and frequent constipation ☐
- Frequent mucus in stool ☐
- Frequent loose stools or diarrhea ☐
- Frequent undigested food in stool ☐
- Fatigue that worsens after eating carbohydrates ☐

NEUROLOGICAL

CHECK ALL THAT APPLY

- Depression ☐
- Brain fog ☐
- Anxiety ☐
- Stress ☐
- Insomnia ☐
- Mood swings ☐
- Frequent irritability ☐
- Fatigue, malaise, or lethargy ☐
- Mental exhaustion ☐
- Trouble concentrating ☐

Frequent forgetfulness ☐

Increased difficulty with memory ☐

Headaches or migraines ☐

Frequent lightheadedness ☐

Frequent fainting ☐

Clumsiness, loss of balance, or lack of coordination ☐

Frequent difficulty speaking distinctly ☐

Moving or speaking slowly ☐

Fidgetiness or restlessness ☐

Tremor or shaky hands ☐

Numbness in hands or feet ☐

Frequent weakness in an arm or a leg ☐

Vertigo or the sensation of the room spinning ☐

Little interest or pleasure in doing things ☐

Decreased satisfaction at work ☐

Deterioration in work performance ☐

Frequent panic attacks ☐

Feeling bad about yourself ☐

Anger management issues ☐

THYROID (HYPERTHYROIDISM)   CHECK ALL THAT APPLY

Fatigue ☐

Feeling jittery, anxious, or nervous ☐

Prone to irritability ☐

Difficulty concentrating ☐

Mood swings ☐

Muscle weakness ☐

Prone to skin rashes ☐

Reduced menstrual flow ☐

Rapid heart rate ☐

Sensitivity to heat ☐

Excessive sweating ☐

Night sweats ☐

Increased appetite ☐

Thinning hair ☐

Dry skin and brittle nails ☐

Diarrhea or loose bowels ☐

Increased thirst ☐

Urinating more often ☐

Sudden weight loss ☐

Difficulty falling asleep ☐

Vision problems ☐

Swelling around face and eyes ☐

Protruding eyes ☐

Dry eyes ☐

Loss of interest in sex ☐

THYROID (HYPOTHYROIDISM)   CHECK ALL THAT APPLY

Hoarseness ☐
Depression ☐
Sluggishness ☐
Insomnia ☐
Thinning hair ☐
Dry skin and brittle nails ☐
Irregular bowel movements ☐
Constipation ☐
Impaired memory ☐
Slowed heart rate ☐
Exhaustion/extreme fatigue ☐
Water retention ☐
Decreased sweating ☐
Increased appetite ☐
Increased thirst ☐
Sugar cravings ☐
Pale, puffy face ☐
Unexplained weight gain ☐
Sensitivity to cold ☐
Cold hands and feet ☐
Numbness or tingling in hands and feet ☐
Elevated blood cholesterol ☐
Irregular or heavy menstrual periods ☐
Muscle weakness, tenderness, and stiffness ☐

JOINTS AND BONES   CHECK ALL THAT APPLY

Sore or swollen joints ☐
Aching or painful muscles ☐
Fatigue and weakness ☐
Fluid in the joints ☐
Loss of mobility ☐
Lack of appetite ☐
Low-grade fever ☐
Stiffness (usually worse in the mornings) ☐
Back pain ☐
Neck pain ☐
Loss in height ☐
Muscle cramps or spasms ☐
Decreased stamina or endurance ☐
Decreased physical strength ☐
Decreased muscle size ☐
Decreased athletic ability ☐
Physical exhaustion ☐

SKIN (INCLUDING LUPUS)   CHECK ALL THAT APPLY

Acne ☐
Rashes ☐
Itching ☐
Hives ☐
Boils ☐
Blisters ☐
Redness ☐
Swelling ☐
Dry or brittle hair ☐
Skin infections ☐
Low-grade fever ☐
Shortness of breath ☐
Athlete's foot ☐
Sensitivity to sun ☐
Discolorations ☐
Scaly patches ☐
Muscle aches ☐
Dry, brittle, or thinning hair ☐
Brittle, peeling, or ridged fingernails ☐
Thinning skin ☐
Dry or scaly skin ☐
Oily skin or hair ☐
Discolored areas of skin ☐
Growths on skin ☐
Scaly, butterfly-shaped rash on face ☐
Dry, scaly lesions on parts of body exposed to sun ☐
Bumps on back of upper arms ☐
Fungus on fingers or toes ☐
Changes in hair or skin texture ☐

ALLERGIES AND SENSITIVITIES   CHECK ALL THAT APPLY

Frequent stuffy ears ☐
Ear pain ☐
Ringing in ears ☐
Hearing loss ☐
Frequent runny nose ☐
Frequent nosebleeds ☐
Sinus pain and infection ☐
Frequent bleeding gums ☐
Hoarseness ☐
Toothache ☐
Frequent sore throat ☐
Pain with swallowing ☐

Frequent trouble swallowing ☐
Frequent or recurrent infections ☐
Frequent wheezing ☐
Frequent coughing ☐
Frequent respiratory infections ☐
Sensitivity to chemicals ☐
Drug allergies ☐
Hypersensitivity to medications, foods, environments, etc. ☐
Allergy or sensitivity to aerosols (fragrance, smoke, cleaning products) ☐
Allergy or sensitivity to pet dander (dogs, cats, etc.) ☐

DIET

	NO	SOMETIMES	YES
Raised eating fast food, sugary cereals, or commercial frozen dinners	☐	☐	☐
Regularly eat bread, pasta, and other baked goods	☐	☐	☐
Eat highly processed foods	☐	☐	☐
Eat conventionally grown produce (not organic)	☐	☐	☐
Crave sugar, dairy, or baked goods	☐	☐	☐
Eat grilled meats	☐	☐	☐
Eat deli meats	☐	☐	☐
Regularly salt food	☐	☐	☐
Have a sweet tooth	☐	☐	☐
Dislike healthy food	☐	☐	☐
Chew food quickly or not very well	☐	☐	☐
Regularly eat at restaurants	☐	☐	☐
Regularly drink alcohol	☐	☐	☐
Use artificial sweeteners (Splenda, Equal, etc.)	☐	☐	☐
Eat packaged or processed convenience foods	☐	☐	☐
Eat a diet low in fresh, organic fruits and vegetables (less than five servings daily)	☐	☐	☐
Buy packaged foods without checking labels for chemicals and additives	☐	☐	☐

SLEEP

	NO	SOMETIMES	YES
Frequent drowsiness	☐	☐	☐
Sleep less than seven hours each night	☐	☐	☐
Trouble falling asleep	☐	☐	☐
Problems waking in the morning	☐	☐	☐
Wake in the middle of the night	☐	☐	☐
Low energy that interferes with quality of life	☐	☐	☐
Snore	☐	☐	☐
Wake with a headache	☐	☐	☐
Wake feeling tired or not rested	☐	☐	☐
Wake up often throughout the night	☐	☐	☐
Trouble falling back to sleep once awakened	☐	☐	☐
Use a sleep apnea device	☐	☐	☐

Take herbal or over-the-counter medication to sleep   ☐   ☐   ☐
Take prescription medication to sleep   ☐   ☐   ☐
Told that you stop breathing while asleep   ☐   ☐   ☐
Kick or jerk your legs or arms while asleep   ☐   ☐   ☐
Experience restlessness, tingling, or crawling in your arms or legs   ☐   ☐   ☐

EXERCISE AND WEIGHT CONTROL

	NO	SOMETIMES	YES
Comfortable with current weight	☐	☐	☐
Unexplained weight loss	☐	☐	☐
Unexplained weight gain	☐	☐	☐
Experienced a change in appetite	☐	☐	☐
Consider yourself physically unfit	☐	☐	☐
Exercise less than 150 minutes a week	☐	☐	☐

STRESS

	NO	SOMETIMES	YES
Overeat under stress	☐	☐	☐
Eat too little under stress	☐	☐	☐
Handle stress poorly	☐	☐	☐
Feel you have an excessive amount of stress in your life	☐	☐	☐
Your job is a source of stress	☐	☐	☐
Your family or personal relationships cause you stress	☐	☐	☐
Experienced abuse, a victim of a crime, or had a significant trauma	☐	☐	☐
Hold your emotions in rather than express them	☐	☐	☐
Hold stress in your body	☐	☐	☐
Rarely pray or meditate	☐	☐	☐
Rarely exercise	☐	☐	☐
Experienced major losses in your life	☐	☐	☐

SETTING GOALS

After reviewing your yes answers, do you see a concentration of symptoms in any particular part of the body? List below.

1.
2.
3.

Which areas in your life—such as diet, sleep, exercise, or stress management—look like they could stand improvement? List your ninety-day goals below:

1.
2.
3.
4.
5.

PART I:
AUTOIMMUNITY 101

1

THE SILENT EPIDEMIC

The journey of a thousand miles begins with a single step.

– Lao Tzu

The shuffling, zombie-like person at the grocery store, the overweight woman with thinning hair, the mom who is always too tired to spend time with her kids, the professional who spends every spare moment sleeping—please don't judge them and brand them as lazy, fat, or apathetic. Chances are they're ill and barely able to accomplish everyday tasks. Although men are affected to a lesser degree than women, they can struggle with the same seemingly inexplicable symptoms.

Because those living with autoimmunity may not be visibly ill, many people don't view them as actually sick. Even their own doctors, co-workers, partners, and loved ones may dismiss their symptoms since they're not readily apparent.

Autoimmunity ("auto," meaning self, and "immunity," meaning protection) develops when your immune system misidentifies your body's healthy tissues as foreign intruders and launches an attack. Autoimmune disease can exist undetected for decades, doing its dirty work out of the spotlight, gradually and quietly. The autoimmune disease you develop depends on which tissues your immune system attacks. Target areas can include organs, glands, joints, muscles, skin, connective tissue, blood vessels, red blood cells, and compounds such as hormones and enzymes.

Over time, chronic responses can manifest as celiac disease, rheumatoid arthritis, multiple sclerosis, asthma, lupus, diabetes, or a host of other autoimmune disorders. Even seemingly unrelated conditions such as depression, obesity, neurological disorders, and certain types of cancer can be traced back to systemic inflammatory responses.

Your immune system is designed to attack and destroy viruses, bacteria, parasites, toxins, and other invaders. When it encounters threats beyond the threshold of its capability, it can go haywire. Unlike our ancestors, modern humans are barraged with a dizzying array of foreign invaders, including many that didn't exist a mere century ago. Our immune systems have to contend with plastic food containers, chemical pesticides on produce, car exhaust, air fresheners, laundry detergents, cosmetics, hair dyes, food additives (even in all-natural and organic foods), and genetic tinkering in the food supply. All of these add up.

Much like how an ancient army would be no match for drones and bombs, our immune system is not equipped to battle modern-day toxins. It cannot effectively defend the body against things like chemical compounds that bind to the thyroid, heavy metals that morph with DNA, or processed foods like wheat engineered beyond recognition.

THE BACKSTORY

Autoimmune diseases have been on the rise for the past fifty years. This is not a result of more awareness but rather an actual increase in the number of people affected. According to the American Autoimmune Related Diseases Association (AARDA), 10 percent of the world's population, including 52 million Americans, are living with some form of autoimmune disease—and that number is rapidly growing.

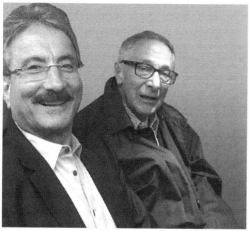

Autoimmunity used to be considered rare. In 1898, Nobel Prize–winning German immunologist Paul Ehrlich coined the term "horror autotoxicus" (literally, "the horror of self-toxicity") to describe his theory that the human body would not attack itself. This mindset persisted in the scientific community until 1956, when pioneering American scientist Noel R. Rose was able to reproduce Hashimoto's thyroiditis (one of over 100 recognized autoimmune diseases) in rabbits by injecting them with thyroglobulin, a protein naturally produced by the thyroid gland. Rose's revolutionary experiments revealed that the animals produced an immune response that inflamed and destroyed their own thyroid glands. Worried about challenging conventional wisdom, Rose worked with fellow scientist and mentor Ernest Witebsky on several more experiments until they had undeniable scientific evidence that

The late Noel R. Rose, MD, PhD, pioneered the modern era of research into autoimmune disease. His contributions to the field are numerous and nothing short of monumental. He's pictured here (right) with my father at a medical conference they attended together in 2016.

the body, under hostile circumstances, could actually turn against itself. Today, Rose is recognized as the father of autoimmune disease research.

After Rose and Witebsky jointly published their findings in several medical journals, a bright young research assistant in England named Deborah Doniach reached out to the pair. She wondered whether Hashimoto's could possibly be an autoimmune disease. This exchange of ideas led to Doniach publishing her own articles with immunologist Ivan Roitt.

As more articles about autoimmunity began to surface, Ehrlich's long-held dictum concerning the body's natural aversion to self-destruction was turned upside down. For the next ten years, between 1955 and 1965, the scientific community debated whether autoimmunity actually existed, and the concept gradually gained acceptance among more researchers. Even as the medical community caught on, however, they failed to grasp the bigger picture: Autoimmunity is an immune issue specific to no particular tissue, gland, or organ, but is the common denominator in multiple diseases.

In the 1970s, physicians rushed to claim autoimmune disease subspecialties, such as joints, neurological tissue, or the digestive tract, instead of addressing immune dysfunction as a broader, systemic problem.

Meanwhile, the industrial chemical revolution was well underway, quietly and insidiously taking root in day-to-day life. Production plants sprang up across the United States, churning out synthetic goods such as plastics, flame retardants, body products, artificial food additives, toxic household cleaners, Teflon compounds, pesticides, insecticides, herbicides—the list is endless. This incremental rise in toxic substances in our environment has contributed to the significant rise of autoimmune diseases. Studies consistently reveal that chemicals and heavy metals can trigger autoimmunity by disrupting hormones and binding to tissues so that the immune system can no longer distinguish friend from foe.

HOW THE INDUSTRIAL CHEMICAL REVOLUTION GAVE RISE TO AUTOIMMUNITY

Our bodies are a microcosm of the planet, made up of the very minerals, trace elements, and microbes that constitute Earth itself. We do not exist separately from the natural world; rather, we are as rooted in it as the plants, trees, mountains, and oceans. Our entire genetic makeup is the result of billions of years of evolution. Since the first *Homo sapiens* (modern humans) emerged 300,000 years ago, we've adapted to our surroundings and thrived by consuming organic and carbon-based foods. In less than a century, all that changed.

Sadly, our relationship with the planet has become more and more detached, with environmental factors accounting for 70 percent of all autoimmune diseases. Many of us are old enough to remember a time when food allergies and sensitivities were uncommon and when autism, type 1 diabetes, and multiple sclerosis were relatively rare. Upticks in these and other ailments have led researchers to take a closer look at what is making so many of us ill. Not surprisingly, the evidence points to environmental factors, generally divided into chemicals, modified foods, and pathogens (bacteria, viruses, or other microorganisms).

In recent decades, we've bombarded our environment and food supply with more than 80,000 synthetic chemicals. Even more disturbing is that less than 5 percent of these man-made compounds have been tested for human toxicity. Meanwhile, an average of 2,500 new chemicals are introduced each year. Currently, there are 6 million chemical-laced products made for human use that cannot be metabolized, causing the toxins to accumulate in body tissues. This is known as the body burden of chemicals.

The standard American diet is filled with preservatives, food dyes, gums, thickening agents, flavorings, meat glues, and genetically modified plants and animals. Even many foods labeled "organic" contain substances that didn't exist fifty years ago. In an effort to boost profits, food manufacturers have toyed with plant genetics, refined and processed our traditional foods, and combined chemicals that have manufactured entirely new protein structures. The human body is simply unable to adapt to the rapid pace of these changes.

Until a century or so ago, food comprised lipids, carbohydrates, proteins, and nucleic acids. Now, our food is grown with pesticides, insecticides, fungicides, and artificial fertilizers, and livestock is treated with antibiotics and hormones and may even be given contaminated feed. Food travels along conveyor belts and through factory tubing before being packaged in synthetic material, all of which expose it to toxic chemicals. The end result is food that contains an astonishing amount of synthetic substances.

Consider the journey beef takes before it ends up on your plate. Like most food manufacturers, factory farmers are focused on the bottom line. To increase profits, they raise cows en masse and crowd them into tight spaces. To plump them up fast, the cows are given hormone shots. Disease can run rampant under these conditions, so the cows are given antibiotics, too. Finally, most of these cows are malnourished because they are fed corn instead of freely grazing on grass in a pasture. After slaughter, the meat is injected with nitrates and other chemicals, then wrapped in plastic before being transported. All of this is a far cry from the hunt-and-eat method of our ancestors.

Even the simple wheat consumed for thousands of years is now offered to us in a newfangled, hybridized form. Today's wheat is sprayed with chemical pesticides and cultivated in polluted, nutrient-deficient soil, and then goes through lengthy processing, packaging, and preserving before ever reaching your table.

Fundamentally, we eat to absorb the vital nutrients needed to survive and thrive. As an incentive to facilitate this necessary and life-sustaining process, food consumption is generally pleasurable. Beyond that, food helps connect us to our bodies, family and friends, community, and heritage. Individually, we need to make decisions about what we consume that affects our health, wellness, and planet. This book is designed to arm you with the information you need to make the choices that can change your autoimmunity.

WHAT CONVENTIONAL DOCTORS WILL TELL YOU

Western medicine fails to address that autoimmunity can be silently underway for years before the symptoms appear. As an example, over 20 million Americans have thyroid disease, an autoimmune disorder, and 60 percent of them don't know they have it. Labs may even conclude that someone's test results are within the acceptable range, so that patient's complaints are often dismissed.

The average doctor visit typically lasts sixteen minutes—hardly enough time to examine a patient's lifestyle and eating habits. In addition to being rushed, many conventional doctors follow outdated information, prescribe medications to mask symptoms, and are unable to recognize autoimmunity. By the time a patient receives a diagnosis, their autoimmune disease has run rampant. Once officially diagnosed, patients are given prescription medications that fail to address the root cause of the illness. In fact, few—if any—doctors will ask about your diet. Eczema? They'll tell you it's due to the climate. Rheumatoid arthritis? They'll chalk it up to old age. The majority of patients I see in my practice have gone from doctor to doctor looking for answers.

Autoimmune disease comes in different forms and in varying degrees of severity. More than 100 different diseases fall under the umbrella of autoimmunity, which explains why many conventional doctors fail to understand that the same issue underlies all of them: an immune system gone haywire. It's hard to fathom that the driver behind your chronic diarrhea (gastrointestinal autoimmunity), for instance, is essentially the same thing causing your angry red skin outbreaks (psoriasis).

WHAT A FUNCTIONAL IMMUNOLOGIST WILL TELL YOU

Functional medicine practitioners focus on getting to the root cause of medical conditions by examining the patient's lifestyle and entire history. If you have one or more autoimmune diseases, lifestyle choices can significantly improve your health and diminish the effects of your illness. Forty-five percent of autoimmune patients are labeled as hypochondriacs by doctors in the early stages of their disease.

Women represent 75 to 80 percent of people living with autoimmune diseases. Unfortunately, we still haven't advanced to the point where all physicians take women's concerns and emotions seriously. In fact, women are far more susceptible to allergic disorders, autoimmune diseases, migraines, and irritable bowel syndrome due to a combination of mast cells (which differ from men's) and hormones, which are more complex and fluctuate more than men's.

In addition, a "healthy" diet might not be what it seems. The links between autoimmune disease and gluten, dairy casein, and lectins (found in legumes, grains, and nightshade vegetables) have been scientifically proven. High levels of sugar and dietary sodium have also been shown to affect the immune system, as have low levels of vitamin D. Historically, diets were high in vitamin D and people were outside getting enough sun exposure to trigger the body to create vitamin D. Now, many people eat nutrient-poor diets and spend most of their time indoors.

The National Institutes of Health (NIH) conducted a study in 2005 on twins and found that heredity could only account for the development of about one-third of all autoimmune diseases. That means autoimmune disease can develop without a genetic component.

Take celiac disease, for example. Certain variants of the HLA-DQA1 and HLA-DBQB1 genes play a critical role in the development of the disease, but only 10 percent of all patients with the genetic predisposition develop celiac disease. Conversely, many people end up with celiac disease without having the genes.

Persistent infection can also drive autoimmunity. If the immune system never perceives that it has cleared an infection 100 percent, it will continue to produce more and more antibodies. Over the course of years, this constant strain on the immune system can develop into an autoimmune condition.

Chronic stress is another contributing factor. Troubled relationships, negative social interactions, demanding careers, loneliness, and lack of sleep have all been linked to increases in pro-inflammatory responses.

Leaky gut syndrome, also known as increased intestinal permeability, allows harmful molecules to penetrate from the intestinal tract into the circulatory system. This is one of the leading causes driving autoimmunity and food immune reactivity.

Despite all these factors, autoimmunity can often be mitigated with little or no medicine. Depending on how far the disease has progressed, it might only take a few simple dietary and lifestyle changes to place it into remission.

It's important to note that normal laboratory test results don't tell the whole story. Standard lab tests are usually based on population averages, which means your results are formulated based on their relation to test results from a control base of healthy people. If your symptoms persist despite "normal" lab results, a functional medicine doctor will continue to run tests to determine the root cause.

The growing number of people with autoimmune diseases is a sign of what's to come for a significant portion of our population if everyone—doctors included—continues to accept "normal" lab results as the bottom line.

The good news is, there are answers. Through science, we can pinpoint the contributing factors to each patient's unique autoimmunity. Once we know the cause(s), we can develop a road map back to better health.

THERE IS NO ONE SINGLE ANSWER

Autoimmunity is complex and is almost never traced to a solitary trigger. A combination of factors can include:

- Genetics
- Infections
- Lifestyle
- Environment
- Diet—the top contributing factor to autoimmunity

By reading this book, you are already taking a significant step in reclaiming your health by learning about autoimmunity, including how it develops, what you can do to take control of your condition, and how to heal using the Detect-Remove-Repair protocol.

STAGES OF AUTOIMMUNITY

First, the immune system mistakenly targets healthy tissue with antibodies. Antibodies then signal the immune system to attack and destroy the targeted tissue. Some types of autoimmunity may be caused by a leftover inflammatory response from the body fighting cancer. A body injury may also play a role in some autoimmune diseases, because the immune system may attack healthy tissue while trying to heal internal wounds, resulting in inflammation of the joints and tendons.

Most autoimmune diseases can go completely unnoticed for many years before symptoms develop. This is the stage of silent autoimmunity, or what I like to call the "ignition," when you are asymptomatic but autoimmunity has begun. During this stage, the only clues are elevations in antibody levels. As a preventive measure, we can now test for predictive antibodies before symptoms begin to manifest. Predictive antibodies indicate that autoimmunity may be occurring and there is an increased risk of disease. The results of these predictive tests can also reveal susceptibility to autoimmunity so you can avoid this stage in the first place.

The second stage of autoimmunity is autoimmune reactivity, or the "flame." This occurs when the disease has progressed far enough that general lab tests will show positive results. At this stage, there may be loss of function in certain parts of the body. This can, depending on the disease, include brain fog, eczema, unexplained weight gain, and more. Because these symptoms are vague, however, doctors may miss the signs and not consider testing.

The final stage is active autoimmune disease, or the "wildfire." This is when symptoms can no longer be denied, lab tests are usually positive, and tissue damage and loss of function are so extreme that glands and organs no longer work properly. Fingers can't grasp, legs have difficulty walking, and eyesight is growing dimmer. All too often at this stage, when the disease is undeniably clinically diagnosable, quality of life has already been severely compromised. This is why it's critical to catch the process early, and why testing for predictive antibodies is vital in preventing, halting, or potentially reversing the course of an autoimmune disease.

AUTOIMMUNE DISEASES AND DISORDERS

Today, we know of more than 100 documented autoimmune disorders. This staggering number has put a spotlight on autoimmunity and led to numerous studies that attribute a malfunctioning immune system as the main cause. Here are some of the better known autoimmune disorders.

- Addison's disease
- Ankylosing spondylitis (AS)
- Attention deficit disorder (ADD)
- Attention deficit/hyperactivity disorder (ADHD)
- Celiac disease
- Chronic inflammatory demyelinating polyneuropathy (CIDP)
- Crohn's disease
- Dermatitis herpetiformis (DH)
- Dermatomyositis
- Discoid lupus erythematosus (DLE)
- Eczema
- Glomerulonephritis
- Graves' disease
- Guillain-Barré syndrome
- Hashimoto's thyroiditis
- Hidradenitis suppurativa
- Idiopathic urticaria
- Irritable bowel syndrome (IBS)
- Inflammatory bowel disease (IBD)
- Juvenile idiopathic arthritis
- Lichen planus
- Multiple sclerosis (MS)
- Myasthenia gravis
- Neuromyelitis optica (NMO)
- Obsessive-compulsive disorder (OCD)
- Parkinson's disease
- Pernicious anemia
- Psoriasis
- Psoriatic arthritis (PsA)
- Reactive arthritis
- Rheumatoid arthritis (RA)
- Scleroderma
- Small intestinal bacterial overgrowth (SIBO)
- Sjögren's syndrome
- Spondyloarthritis (SpA)
- Systemic lupus erythematosus (SLE)
- Systemic sclerosis (SSc)
- Type 1 diabetes
- Ulcerative colitis
- Vitiligo

The next important step is finding a qualified practitioner. They should be experienced and knowledgeable about autoimmunity and functional medicine, have your best health in mind, and be comfortable interpreting laboratory testing. If you need help finding a practitioner, start at the Institute of Functional Medicine, a global leader in twenty-first century medicine. Visit them online at IFM.org to search for certified practitioners in your area.

Finally, it's crucial to remember that many people are successfully managing their autoimmunity and you can, too. You'll learn how to avoid processed foods, artificial chemical additives, toxic household cleaning products, body products laden with chemicals, and synthetic scents like those found in dryer sheets, fragrances, and air fresheners.

Reclaiming your health also involves reining in your stress levels and learning how to navigate a frenzied American lifestyle. Pace yourself, put your own needs first, and say no when necessary. It's OK to rest and release toxic, draining, and meaningless relationships. You will learn to live with a gentle purpose guided by wisdom and respect for your body's needs.

2

THE IMMUNE SYSTEM

It is health that is real wealth and not pieces of gold and silver.

– Mahatma Gandhi

The immune system is made up of a complex army of cells, chemicals, and organs charged with protecting your body from invading toxins and pathogens. Without it, you wouldn't be able to survive the conditions of modern life, and even the smallest of perils—a splinter, a stubbed toe, or an accidental slice of the finger while chopping vegetables—could be life-threatening. But white blood cells are already at the site, quickly, quietly, and mightily sending chemical signals to the rest of the immune system, already working to protect you from infection before you even have time to stick on a bandage.

We can divide the immune system into two parts: innate and adaptive. Innate immunity is present in your body since birth, while adaptive immunity is acquired over the course of a lifetime, adapting to new infections through the creation of antibodies. Innate immunity is sometimes called "non-specific," while adaptive immunity is called "specific."

Your innate immunity targets anything it perceives as foreign, meaning it is non-specific in its mission to seek out and destroy invaders. As your body's first line of defense, your innate immunity relies on inflammatory cytokines released by T-helper cell types 1 (Th1) and 17 (Th17), as well as others.

Adaptive immunity, on the other hand, is exceedingly specific, sending out specialized antibodies for a particular antigen it has previously encountered. Whenever you get vaccinated for the flu, for example, you are enlisting your adaptive immunity to create antibodies for that specific antigen.

THE MAKING OF AN IMMUNE SYSTEM

Every human life begins the same way, with a single-cell sperm penetrating the outer layer of a single-cell egg. Together, the sperm and egg form a completely new single-cell organism informed by billions of years of evolutionary history. In the womb, that single cell divides and multiplies, growing from zygote

KNOW YOUR IMMUNE CELLS

Phagocytes are also known as "eating cells." Phagocytes include two subtypes—**macrophages** and **neutrophils**. Think of them collectively as the Pac-Man of the immune system, gobbling up harmful organisms and infected cells as they circulate through the body.

Mast cells and basophils are a class of white blood cells typically responsible for inflammatory responses to allergens. Mast cells release histamine and live in the mucosal lining of the sinuses, throat, lungs, and digestive tract, while basophils are designed to fight parasitic infections but can also be involved in allergic reactions.

Natural killer (NK) cells are another type of white blood cell that targets tumors and body cells infected with pathogens.

Eosinophils are inflammatory white blood cells that target larger pathogens like parasitic worms. They're also responsible for allergic responses.

Dendritic cells act as messengers to other cells. They become increasingly more important once the adaptive immune system develops.

B cells attack pathogens situated outside of body cells. They also act as a cleanup crew after T cells go on the attack. We'll talk more about B cells and their specialized antibodies (called immunoglobulins) in Chapter 4.

T cells target a specific antigen from inside an infected cell and can only attack if signaled by other immune cells, typically dendritic cells or macrophages. T cells come in three main types:

- **Killer T cells**, also known as cytotoxic T cells, bind to antigens displayed on infected cells and release messenger proteins called cytokines. Cytokines open the pores of a diseased cell so it can be eaten by a macrophage.
- **Regulatory T cells (Tregs)** act as the immune system's police force, patrolling the circulatory system, supporting immune homeostasis, and inducing tolerance between friendly bacteria and food antigens.

to embryo to fetus. DNA inside embryonic cells (also known as stem cells) is busy turning on and off genes, providing instructions to develop into one of about 200 different types of specialized cells, including those that will go on to form organs such as the brain, heart, and kidneys. Over the course of several months, some cells will go on to become immune cells, or part of the innate immune system.

At birth, we transition from the sterile environment of our mother's womb into a world teeming with bacteria, viruses, and toxins. If we arrive via vaginal birth, we're covered in diverse microbes on our way out; these organisms will colonize our guts and skin, establishing our microbiome and activating our adaptive immune system. Babies born by Cesarean section are introduced to a different set of microbes—from the air, the nurses in the maternity ward, and whatever else might be in the environment. We are all born with no antibodies and an immature immune system.

Antibodies from breast milk also spark the adaptive immune system, which continues to develop as we encounter new microbes in our environment. Beginning at about three months of age, stem cells in bone marrow start forming two special types of white blood cells. B cells remain in the bone marrow until they mature and then migrate to the spleen and lymph nodes. T cells migrate to the thymus while they are still immature. In the thymus, T cells are put through a rigorous bootcamp that forces them to recognize "self" antigens from "non-self" antigens. Cells that fail this rigorous testing—and most do—are destroyed in the thymus. Those that do pass leave the thymus to enter the circulatory system.

White blood cells are the cornerstone of the immune system. When activated by an intruding antigen, B and T cells produce highly specialized antibodies that remember foreign invaders after just one exposure. Should that particular invader return, the specialized B and T cells will recognize it and spring into action to fight it off.

At the same time, we are also developing our lymphatic system, a vital part of the immune system consisting of thin tubes known as lymph vessels and oval-shaped tissues called lymph nodes. Lymph vessels carry lymph fluid, which serves as a cell waste collection system and helps distribute immune cells throughout the body. Lymph nodes, on the other hand, contain white blood cells that filter the lymph fluid. When your doctor examines your lymph nodes for swelling (an indication of a sickness), it's to see if your immune system is in overdrive.

TOLERANCE LEVELS

Our guts begin to populate with good bacteria during infancy, creating something called central tolerance—a mechanism that trains immune system cells to differentiate between "self" and "non-self" tissue and prevents attacking anything it identifies as self. This happens in a walnut-sized organ called the thymus, located just above the heart, and takes about two or three years to fully develop. Since our environment is ever changing, our immune system has to keep up as we adapt to new things. This is where peripheral tolerance comes into play. Peripheral tolerance happens in the gut and, like central tolerance, tries to discern self from non-self but with more flexibility.

Oral tolerance is a subtype of peripheral tolerance. Each time you take a bite of food, you challenge your immune system to recognize whether proteins in that food are enemies. At the same time, your immune system is checking for harmful microbes. Oral tolerance is the suppression of an immune response against harmless elements in the food we eat. Without it, your body would launch an allergic attack every time you ate.

Autoimmunity causes people to suddenly start reacting to certain foods for the first time. This is called loss of oral tolerance, which causes your body to no longer be able to identify certain foods as safe. It's also a clear indication that your immune system is misfiring, mistaking healthy tissue as a threat and attacking.

THE HYGIENE HYPOTHESIS

The premise of the hygiene hypothesis is that a child who lives with siblings or regularly plays with other children will be exposed to numerous types of bacteria, viruses, and other harmful elements. This exposure helps their immune system learn how to effectively fight off things that will cause illness. By comparison, a child who never gets dirty and lives in a relatively sterile environment won't gain certain immunity advantages and will have difficulty battling infections as an adult.

While this hypothesis is widely believed, it hasn't been proven entirely accurate. The paper that inspired it, "Hay Fever, Hygiene, and Household Size," was written

- **T-helper (Th) cells** release inflammatory cytokines and stimulate B cells to make more antibodies. T-helper cells fall into specific subtypes, including Th1, Th2, Th3, Th9, Th17, or TFH. All of these facilitate distinct types of cytokines and immune responses.

- **Th1 cells** are part of the innate immune system that causes an inflammatory response in the presence of an invader. This is what causes pus to surround a splinter in your finger, for example.

- **Th2 cells**, or "memory cells," are the linchpins of adaptive immunity and the basis for vaccines. If a foreign antigen enters the body, Th2 cells communicate with B cells, which in turn produce antibodies that will recognize that same antigen in future invasions and counter with a stronger, more accurate response. A balance between Th1 and Th2 response is necessary for the immune system to achieve homeostasis.

- **Th3 cells** also participate in the maintenance of immune homeostasis.

- **Th17 cells** are so called because they produce interleukin-17 cytokines. They also produce the signaling cytokines interleukin-6, interleukin-21, interleukin 23, and transforming growth factor beta (TGF-ß). Normally, Th17 cells provide antimicrobial immunity in mucosal barriers.

- **Follicular T-helper cells (TFH)** are formed by the interleukin-21 cytokine.

NOTES FROM THE LAB

Over the course of a lifetime, your immune system will develop the capacity to create up to a quintillion distinct antibodies. A quintillion is a million trillions, or a one followed by eighteen zeroes.

in 1989 by an epidemiologist named David P. Strachan, out of the London School of Hygiene and Tropical Medicine. It states that kids do better under germy conditions because T-helper cells type 1 (Th1) get more rigorous training in early life, which potentially reduces the risk of developing allergies. (Cytokines produced by T-helper cells type 1 are responsible for allergic responses.)

While the hygiene hypothesis and the origin of allergic responses is still a hotly debated topic among researchers, it doesn't explain the rise of autoimmune diseases mediated by T-helper cells type 1.

In 2003, a group of immunologists including Graham Rook, a professor of medical microbiology at the University College London, provided an alternative theory in a paper titled "Old Friends Hypothesis." Rook suggests that early and regular exposure to the ancient microorganisms that co-evolved with us for thousands of years are what actually strengthen our immunity. This includes the microbes in mud, gardens, animals—anything that exposes us to the natural world.

Humans used to live in dwellings made from mud, timber, and thatch. Our guts, or "ancient microbiome," reflected these environs and were populated by many of the same microbes found in these natural materials. Today, however, we live in sterile, insulated homes made from biocide-treated timber, plasterboard, and plastics.

The old friends hypothesis states that regular, frequent exposure to beneficial natural microorganisms at a young age trains the immune system to produce more regulatory T cells, or Tregs.

TREGS AND THE DELICATE BALANCE OF T-HELPER CELLS

When functioning properly, the innate and adaptive immune systems work together to protect the body from invading pathogens. While this often entails inflammation, regulatory T cells, or Tregs, step in to suppress and regulate inflammation once the pathogens are successfully obliterated. Without Tregs, T-helper cells would produce too many cytokine responses, resulting in overinflammation and tissue damage. Tregs also instruct the friendly bacteria in our gastrointestinal tracts to live in harmony with the foods we eat daily. This is how oral tolerance develops.

In short, Tregs police the immune system and prevent cytokine storms, or hypercytokinemia, which can be life-threatening. If the immune system is under constant threat and in a continuous state of inflammation, Tregs lose their ability to properly regulate T-helper cells when they go on the defense. Harmful gut bacteria, a diet rich in processed foods, environmental chemicals, sickness, infection, stress, a heated argument, overexercising, blood sugar crashes, and lack of sleep are just some of the many examples that can induce an onslaught of cytokines.

Cytokines are hormonal messenger cells produced by a number of different immune cells, most notably T cells. Like T cells, cytokines come in different varieties—interferon, interleukin, and chemokines, to name a few. The wrong kind of cytokines can throw the body out of its desired state of homeostasis, where all systems are stable and in balance.

Maintaining the delicate balance of immune homeostasis is also reflected in the relationship between type 1 and type 2 T-helper cells. Each secretes distinct cytokines: T-helper 1 cells react to pathogens and cancer cells, and T-helper 2s react to parasites. In a healthy immune system, the two are balanced and switch back and forth between responses.

However, when there's an imbalance between them and the cytokines they produce, it can lead to overinflammation and getting "stuck" in one response—meaning too much T-helper 1 or too much T-helper 2. As a result, the immune system begins to attack harmless substances (which leads to allergies) or self-antigens (which leads to autoimmunity). This also holds true for imbalances between T-helper 3 and T-helper 17 cells. When an immune imbalance renders Tregs dysfunctional, the normally protective T-helper 17 cells turn against the body. This contributes to the pathogenesis—meaning the origination and development—of multiple autoimmune diseases, including allergic inflammation, rheumatoid arthritis, autoimmune gastritis, inflammatory bowel disease, psoriasis, and multiple sclerosis. T-helper 1 and T-helper 17 together contribute to systemic autoimmune processes.

As we just noted, Tregs play a key role in keeping the immune system in balance by suppressing inflammation. Most Tregs reside in the gut and possibly have the ability to control the development of allergies, hypersensitivities, and autoimmune diseases. If the immune system is in a constant inflammatory mode because of outside stressors, however, Tregs lose their ability to regulate the immune system—allowing for an imbalance of cytokine responses that ignite the fire.

ANTIGENS AND ANTIBODIES

On the surface of every plant and animal cell are proteins called antigens, which can be divided into two distinct categories: self antigens and non-self antigens. Self antigens thinly coat every cell in your body and act as biomarkers that identify themselves as part of you. On the flip side, non-self antigens originate outside the body and are found in the foods we eat and on the surface of pathogens.

The structure of any given antigen depends on the cell or pathogen. For example, antigens on a flu virus will look different from antigens in a bacterial infection. Think of an antigen as a unique tag that announces its presence, whether as a general "I'm part of you," or "I'm a friendly food," or a specific "Remember me? I'm that bug you caught last winter." Autoimmunity occurs when your immune system can no longer differentiate between self antigens and foreign non-self antigens.

Your immune system is designed to produce antibodies that tag, remember, identify, and destroy foreign or harmful invaders such as bacteria, viruses, and toxins. Antibodies are basically the Special Forces soldiers of the immune system that swoop into the rescue when you are exposed to a pathogen you've previously encountered. Like antigens, they are highly specialized. For example, the antibodies used to fight off the flu will differ from the antibodies that activate the release of histamines to combat an allergy.

SIGNS OF A WEAKENED IMMUNE SYSTEM

- Stress
- Fatigue
- Frequent colds and infections
- Digestive issues
- Slow-healing wounds

THE DIGESTIVE SYSTEM

Life would not long remain possible in the absence of microbes.

– Louis Pasteur

The digestive system acts as a physical barrier in very much the same manner as the external skin. In fact, the GI tract is lined with internal skin. Think of it as a long, fleshy tube that starts in the mouth and ends at the rectum. When all is well, a healthy digestive system allows food to pass through the body without actually entering the body.

The digestive journey is basically a series of processes that break food down into nutrients to be absorbed or waste to be eliminated. It begins even before you take your first bite as your salivary glands secrete saliva in anticipation of receiving food. As you chew, enzymes in your saliva mix with the food and break it down into smaller particles. When you swallow, the chewed food travels down the esophagus to the stomach.

About the size of a boxing glove, your stomach continues to break down the food through a series of muscular contractions and powerful digestive juices called hydrochloric acid and pepsin. Most likely, some harmful microbes hitched a ride on your meal, so your digestive juices seek to kill those off, too. Roughly speaking, each meal spends around four or five hours in the stomach, where it is reduced to a frothy liquid called acidic chyme (pronounced "kime") in preparation for its journey to the small intestine, where nutrients will get absorbed.

After passing through the stomach, the chyme travels through the twists and turns of about twenty-two feet of intestinal tubing and is chemically broken down even further into simple molecules. The liver sends bile to break down the fats, and then the pancreas sends enzyme-rich juices called lipase, protease, and amylase to reduce starches into glucose and fat molecules into fatty acids. Proteins are broken down into peptides (a chain of two or more amino acids) that are then reduced to individual amino acids.

As tiny molecules, the nutrients are now small enough to be absorbed through the intestinal wall and transported through the bloodstream to the lymphatic vessels and ultimately the rest of the body.

What's not absorbed at this stage is pushed through to the large intestine, where water and salts are absorbed into the body. Billions of gut microbes happily feast on what the small intestine rejects, which is mostly fiber. Also called the colon, the large intestine sends whatever remains to its final destination, the rectum. The last leg of the digestive journey ends when the remaining waste is eliminated as you go to the bathroom.

When your diet and gut are healthy, this system works harmoniously, with your digestive system removing what it needs from foods and discarding the rest. Unfortunately, stress, medications, processed foods, lack of digestive enzymes, chemicals in our foods, and other environmental factors can impact this delicate balance and decrease your ability to properly break down all the foods you eat. As a result, your gut and the immune system must grapple with undigested fats, proteins, and carbohydrates, opening the door to food immune reactivity, molecular mimicry, and leaky gut.

LEAKY GUT: THE GATEWAY TO AUTOIMMUNITY

The small intestine really isn't small. Uncoiled, it runs about twenty-two feet and is lined with a single layer of protective cells called the epithelial layer, which separates the gut from the bloodstream. (Incidentally, epithelial cells are similar to the cells that cover the skin on our hands and face, and are renewed every three or four days.) The epithelial layer comprises villi (tiny, hairlike projections that facilitate the passage of fluids and nutrients) and proteins called tight junctions, which "cement" the epithelial cells together. Tight junctions work like microscopic doors that selectively open to allow water and nutrients into the bloodstream and close to block anything harmful. Think of them as the bouncers of the gut, picking and choosing who they want to let in. This is called intestinal permeability, and without it, our bodies would not be able to deliver nutrients to the body.

The terms intestinal permeability and intestinal barrier are often used interchangeably, but they're actually vastly different things. While permeability relates to how easily substances pass through the intestinal wall, the barrier (or gut barrier) is the gut wall. In addition to epithelial cells, villi, and tight junctions, the gut wall also consists of a mucosal layer that protects its from whatever flows through the GI tract. It's one of the body's largest mucosal areas, equivalent to the size of two tennis courts and requiring approximately 40 percent of the body's energy output.

Increased intestinal permeability is another medical term worth knowing. It's used to describe an overly porous, leaky gut. In short, leaky gut results when the epithelial layer is damaged and tight junctions are compromised by inflammation. Gaps in the damaged gut lining allow all manner of macromolecules—food proteins, bacteria, yeast, and other toxic compounds—into the bloodstream where they don't belong. When this happens, the immune system perceives these macromolecules as foreign invaders and launches an attack. This triggers an ever worsening cycle of inflammation throughout the body, which damages the gut, which causes more inflammation, which then damages the gut, leading to an endless cycle.

Depending on your genetic predisposition, leaky gut can result in myriad disorders, including autoimmunity, food immune reactivity, brain fog, depression, chronic pain, joint degeneration, skin disorders, poor nutrition, and more. When it comes to healing leaky gut, microbes matter, because the process starts with fixing your microbiome.

KNOW YOUR MICROBIOME

Imagine the entire 3.7 billion years of evolution compressed into twenty-four hours. That's what Martin J. Blaser, MD, did in his seminal book *Missing Microbes*. As the clock ticks, you'll notice microbes arrive in the first seconds. Our hominid ancestors do not appear until somewhere between forty-seven and ninety-eight seconds before midnight, and we *Homo sapiens* don't arrive on the scene until two seconds before midnight.

But Blaser lists something even more humbling: Despite the fact that millions of microbes (bacteria, viruses, yeast, and fungi) can fit into the eye of a needle, if you were to gather them all together, they would outnumber all the visible life forms we are familiar with, and they would outweigh them as well.

Microbes exist everywhere on this planet—on land, in water, and around all living things. They're wherever the human body is exposed to the outside world—in our mouths, nasal passages, lungs, skin, urogenital tract, and guts. In fact, the vast majority of our "good bugs" live in our guts. This is your microbiome, and it makes up 70 percent of your immune system.

Microbes outnumber us by a lot, even in our own bodies. In 2016, a team of researchers in Israel and Canada concluded that there are 39 trillion bacterial cells for every 30 trillion human cells, a ratio of 1.3 to one.

So microbes, as infinitesimal as they are, are a big deal, at least collectively. Without microbes, we would cease to exist. Take the simple act of breathing, for example. Nitrogen makes up almost four-fifths of the air we inhale, writes Idan Ben-Barak in his enlightening book *The Invisible Kingdom*. But for it to be useful to us, it must be converted to ammonia. Microbes in our respiratory system do that.

We can think of the gut microbiome as a diverse, dynamic garden with its own delicate ecosystem where bacteria, fungi, yeasts, viruses, and archaea form sprawling networks within the colon, growing and interacting like plants in a yard. When these microorganisms stay in balance, the garden thrives. But when the wrong microbes flourish and the "good" microbes starve, it's called gut dysbiosis. When this happens, our "gut garden" suffers, and so does our health. The gut's trillions of microbes aren't simply hitchhikers; they're major modulators of our digestion, nutrient production, and immune function.

Each person's microbiome is a unique product of genetics, lifestyle, and environment, but the foods we eat and the supplements we take can shift its composition, too. Fiber, for instance, stimulates the growth of bacteria that produce short-chain fatty acids (SCFAs)—tiny fats that provide energy to colon cells, help regulate inflammation, and buttress the intestinal wall against invading pathogens. Food additives like emulsifiers, stabilizers, and artificial sweeteners can encourage the growth of harmful bacteria, even helping usher it across

SIGNS YOUR GUT IS LEAKY

Increased intestinal permeability plays a key role in the development of various inflammatory and autoimmune disorders. Some of the signs include:

- Brain fog
- Chronic pain
- Depression
- Fatigue
- Joint degeneration
- Malnutrition
- Skin disorders

NOTES FROM THE LAB

Seventy percent of your immune system resides in your gut. Unfortunately, when the gut breaks down, so does the immune system. Following are some of the proteins that can play a role in the development of leaky gut. We'll be discussing these more in upcoming chapters.

- *Occludin* is an enzyme protein and one of the main component proteins of tight junctions.
- *Actomyosin* is a complex set of proteins that make up muscle fibers and contribute to muscular contractions. If a lab test finds antibodies for actomyosin, it reflects a breakdown of the mucosal lining in the intestinal barrier.
- *Zonulin* is an anchor protein that modulates the permeability of tight junctions. If tight junctions are the bouncers of the gut, zonulin is the doorman who can be bribed into allowing unwanted elements into the premises. Bacterial or chemical toxins can cause zonulin to malfunction, opening the paracellular spaces wide to allow pathogens and oversized protein molecules to enter.

the gut barrier and into the bloodstream. In short, everything we swallow becomes either fertilizer or poison for the garden in our gut.

One of the microbiome's chief functions involves the intestinal barrier—the specialized border separating the body's internal terrain from the external world. It's our first line of defense against antigens and pathogens. Friendly bacteria, which populate the barrier's top layer, help orchestrate the appropriate immune response. When these bacteria encounter antigens from food or harmless organisms, they allow passage through the tight junctions; when they encounter antigens from pathogens, they induce what's called a humoral or cell-mediated response to halt entry. To serve as an effective barrier, the gut mucosal lining must be able to tolerate neutral and beneficial molecules while defending the body against true invaders.

Due to our modern diets, sterilized environments, indoor lifestyles, and use of antibiotics and other bacteria-destroying drugs, human microbiomes today are less diverse than those of our ancestors. This has led to a widespread loss of gut barrier function, increased intestinal permeability, and a breakdown of oral tolerance. As molecules that should be barricaded from entry make their way into circulation, the result is systemwide inflammation, nervous system activation, increased blood-brain barrier permeability, and ultimately a pathway towards brain autoimmunity and neurodegenerative disorders.

PART II:
DETECT THE PROBLEM

4

BE YOUR OWN MEDICAL DETECTIVE

It's like being involved in a detective story, looking for that thing that nobody else has found.

– Erik Larson, mystery writer

Functional medicine experts are a lot like sleuths. When I meet with a new patient, for example, I pore over their medical records, analyze their lab work, ask probing questions, and conduct specialized testing that helps zero in on the root cause behind their health issues. This chapter offers information on how to do some of the detective work yourself.

We'll begin by distinguishing between the three unique classes of food reactivities—allergies, intolerance, and immune reactivity—and the type of testing that should be administered for each. Next, we'll look at the pros and cons of at-home allergy and sensitivity tests, along with those used by conventional doctors. Then we'll dive into the state-of-the-art tests used by functional medicine doctors, followed by an elimination diet plan to follow if testing is not immediately available to you.

DIFFERENCES BETWEEN ALLERGY, INTOLERANCE, AND FOOD IMMUNE REACTIONS

When you go to the doctor because you're reacting to a particular food, you'll likely be given a skin prick test to determine an allergy. The findings will often be negative, and you'll probably leave the office with no clear answers. In fact, many people are tested for allergies when they really should be checked for food immune reactivity. Here's a closer look at the differences.

Food allergies are the result of an immunoglobulin E (IgE) response and tend to trigger serious complications, like anaphylaxis. A classic example is a child with a peanut allergy who immediately reacts to the allergen with hives, wheezing, difficulty breathing, and sometimes sudden death. This is the result of IgE antibodies flooding the body with histamines. Only a few foods—referred to as the Big Eight—are responsible for allergies: milk/dairy, wheat, eggs, peanuts, fish, crustaceans, tree nuts, and soybeans.

Food intolerances are not mediated by the immune system but instead result when the body is unable to break down a particular food properly, usually caused by the absence of certain enzymes. The best-known example is lactose intolerance; people with this condition lack the enzyme lactase. Inflammatory or immune responses are typically less severe than allergies and are mostly restricted to the gastrointestinal tract. Testing for lactose intolerance involves getting a comprehensive stool sample, but most diagnoses are based solely on symptoms, as they tend to be clinically obvious—stomach cramps, pain, nausea, bloating, gas, and diarrhea, for example. Food immune reactions happen anywhere from 1 to 72 hours post consumption.

Food immune reactions are immunoglobulin G (IgG) or immunoglobulin A (IgA) responses controlled by T and B cells. Classic examples include celiac disease and non-celiac gluten sensitivity, unlike food allergies, which cause symptoms immediately, food immune reactions usually occur four to seventy-two hours after exposure. One possibility is leaky gut syndrome, where large protein molecules break through the gut lining and travel into the blood, causing systemic inflammation. Since these antibodies bind to specific food antigens, testing for food immune reactivity involves checking blood for their presence.

AT-HOME ALLERGY AND SENSITIVITY TESTING

You might have seen food sensitivity tests advertised on social media. These kits are ordered online and delivered to your home, where you then prick your finger to draw blood. The blood is then dropped onto a card and mailed to a lab. I've seen firsthand how powerful food immunoglobulin G antibody testing can be when done correctly with the right lab, so I don't blame people for trying to get the information themselves.

That said, I don't recommend these at-home, mail-in tests. They're operated by marketing companies that partner with low-quality food antibody test providers, which means the results are basically meaningless. With food reactivity tests, the purity of the antigen or substrate (a material used for testing) is the most important thing.

These mail-in testing companies use cheap synthetic analogs for the foods they are testing against rather than extracts from actual whole foods. For example, instead of testing against milk peptides—such as pure casein or lactoglobulin, which would mimic how the immune system sees this food as it is digested—these companies test with an artificial protein that resembles whole milk extract.

A high-quality lab will test against proteins extracted directly from food. For instance, if you suspect you have an immune reaction to cod, for instance, the lab should get real cod and extract the proteins to test against. Since heat changes a food's protein structure, the lab should also test for the food in both its raw and cooked state. It's labor-intensive versus just testing with an artificial protein, which takes about a tenth of the time at a twentieth of the cost.

That, in short, is the problem. These companies don't test how the immune system will interact with something in the real world. Unfortunately, many people are so frustrated trying to find answers that they just want to see anything resembling a result.

It's also important to realize that all lab tests have potential for error. This is why I insist on working with laboratories that independently duplicate the initial test to confirm accuracy and also provide pure, high-quality material.

Of course, duplicating a test doubles the cost, so it's not often done in conventional labs, much less the ones used by mail-in testing companies. If a lab can't replicate the results by double testing, then you're susceptible to reporting errors as high as 10 or 15 percent, depending on the technology being used. I recommend asking your medical practitioner about the testing methods of the labs they work with, or ask for the name and call the lab directly. If a lab won't answer your questions, it likely does not double-test or use pure substrates.

STANDARD LABORATORY TESTING

Conventional medicine has its own set of issues, often relying on basic laboratory tests, outdated methods, and poorly designed immunoglobulin G and immunoglobulin A antibody measurements to test for non-immunoglobulin E-mediated food immune reactivity. Moreover, your general practitioner may be out of his or her comfort zone when it comes to interpreting the latest diagnostic tests, so it's wise to seek out a health care professional who is familiar with specialized tests, uses them frequently, and knows how to interpret the results.

The first line of approach when diagnosing food immune reactivity should be a physical examination and a complete evaluation of your medical history, including whether autoimmunity runs in your family. Once you find a specialist and have a thorough consultation about your symptoms, family history, and lifestyle, you can determine which tests are right for you.

Following are some of the standard laboratory tests used by the conventional medical establishment. If you've been going from doctor to doctor trying to figure out why you are feeling unwell, you may already be familiar with some of these.

ALCAT is designed to test for food immune reactivity. It's conducted by adding drops of blood to small amounts of a potential antigen to see if the white blood cells change in size as a "reaction." There are two major problems with this. First, white blood cells may change in size or shape in response to the antigen dropped into the liquid because of the electrical or chemical nature of the protein itself, not because of immune reactions. Second, the reproducibility of the testing has been questioned when split samples have been sent to the same lab.

MRT is essentially the same as ALCAT; it is an alternative version.

LRA (ELISA-ACT) is a third alternative version of ALCAT. It looks at cell reactivity in liquid to different antigens.

Skin prick testing is used to determine a patient's immunoglobulin E-mediated allergies. Small amounts of common food proteins are placed just underneath the skin surface with needles and then the skin is checked for reactions ten to fifteen minutes later. This test looks at the allergic arm of the immune system and has no relationship to food immune reactions and their interplay with autoimmunity. People may also react to impurities in the extracts and not necessarily the actual food. This test is quite reliable for airborne allergens but not for dietary allergens.

KNOW YOUR IMMUNOGLOBULINS

Immunoglobulins are Y-shaped globular proteins produced after your first exposure to a specific bacteria, virus, or toxin. Each type of immunoglobulin serves its own role, and their presence in blood or saliva tests can tell us whether there's a problem.

- ***Immunoglobulin G (IgG)*** accounts for up to 75 percent of the total serum immunoglobulins in your immune system and circulates through your blood and other bodily fluids. IgG protects you from bacteria and viruses, but an overproduction of them can increase permeability of the small intestinal wall, leading to food immune reactions.

- ***Immunoglobulin A (IgA)*** is found primarily in mucosal membranes like the respiratory, urogenital, and gastrointestinal tracts, as well as in saliva, tears, and breast milk. Measuring IgA can determine problems with food immune reactivity. It can also be used to evaluate rheumatoid arthritis, lupus, celiac disease, and kidney and intestinal issues.

- ***Immunoglobulin E (IgE)*** is the least common immunoglobulin isotype but can trigger the most powerful inflammatory and allergic reactions, such as anaphylaxis to peanuts or allergic reactions to pollen or cats. It is found throughout the body, but it's predominantly in the lungs, skin, and mucous membranes. IgE binds to allergens and immediately triggers histamine release from mast cells and basophils, resulting in reactions like hay fever, asthma, and hives. IgE is primarily involved in classic allergic responses, usually to wheat, eggs, peanuts, fish, crustaceans, tree nuts, and soybeans. Measuring IgE levels is also helpful in diagnosing parasitic infections.

- ***Immunoglobulin D (IgD)*** makes up less than 1 percent of antibodies and was discovered in 1964. Its exact function remains unknown, but it is thought to be involved in signaling the production of B cells and playing a part in respiratory immune defense.

- ***Immunoglobulin M (IgM)*** accounts for about 10 percent of the antibodies in the bloodstream and responds to antigen invasions and microbial infections. They are the first antibodies produced and released into the blood about two weeks following an infection. IgM antibodies also present for a specific subtype of leaky gut called endotoxemia.

Patch testing is an alternative to skin prick testing and is less reliable at detecting food allergens than airborne ones.

Immunoglobulin E food allergy testing in blood can be reliable for the identification of classic food allergies.

PREDICTIVE, DIAGNOSTIC, AND IMMUNOLOGICAL LAB WORK

Functional medicine experts like to utilize everything evidence-based science has to offer. We keep an eye on the scientific pipeline and tend to use newer, state-of-the-art tests—such as for leaky gut—ten or fifteen years earlier than our conventional colleagues.

The earlier you can discover your food triggers and genetic predispositions, the sooner you can take charge of your health and prevent years of unnecessary pain. This is where predictive testing comes in. Some of the labs I like to use include Labcorp, Doctor's Data, Quest Diagnostics, and Great Plains Laboratory. (See the Resource section for contact information.) For food sensitivity testing, I use Cyrex Laboratories. Cyrex offers a free one-on-one interpretation with a physician on staff, but most functional and integrative physicians will be familiar with these types of tests and can order them for you. Following is a list of the more common tests we use to detect signs of autoimmunity. All are done with a simple blood test. (Some of these tests might not be available in the state of New York because of its blood testing regulations.)

Array 2: Intestinal Antigenic Permeability Screen. This test identifies leaky gut syndrome and gut dysbiosis (when the bad bacteria outweigh the good) and is recommended for those with a known autoimmune condition, chronic digestive issues, fatigue, or joint pain. It's also recommended for retesting to see whether leaky gut protocols are working. This test looks for antibodies for actomyosin, zonulin, and occludin, the proteins that open tight junctions in the intestinal barrier. It also looks for the presence of endotoxins called lipopolysaccharides (LPS). These large molecules consist of lipids and polysaccharides and are found in the outer membrane of bacteria such as *E. coli* and *H. pylori*. In humans, the presence of lipopolysaccharides triggers an innate immune response, activating the immune system and producing inflammatory cytokines. Together these markers reflect the nature and the degree of gut damage. (Cyrex Laboratories)

Array 3X: Wheat/Gluten Proteome Reactivity and Autoimmunity. Since gluten is the most common trigger for autoimmunity, I often start with this test, which offers the most comprehensive look at non-celiac gluten sensitivity and immune reactivity to other non-gluten components of wheat. It is the gold standard for identifying issues related to gluten consumption. It also checks to see if gluten is impacting the brain. (Cyrex Laboratories)

Array 4: Gluten-Associated Cross-Reactive Foods and Foods Sensitivity. This panel covers non-wheat foods including dairy, corn, soy, eggs, and most gluten-free grain replacements such as buckwheat, amaranth, corn, rice, potato, tapioca, and quinoa. If you are going to start a gluten-free diet based on your blood testing, it's important to be sure you don't replace gluten with another food that you are equally reactive to. This panel covers the most common foods that may present that risk. (Cyrex Laboratories)

Array 5: Multiple Autoimmune Reactivity Screen. This looks for antibodies to multiple antigens in one test. Because it measures predictive antibodies up to ten years before the clinical onset of a disease, it's a great way to determine whether an autoimmune process is silently at work. It is recommended for those in the initial stages of autoimmune conditions who are experiencing joint pain, fatigue, brain fog, memory loss, hair loss, or unusual weight gain or loss. The test looks for autoimmunity against the brain, joints, adrenal gland, thyroid gland, liver, platelets, intestines, and heart, and is helpful in pinpointing the cause and location of the underlying problem, along with the specificity of further tests to take. (Cyrex Laboratories)

Array 7: Neurological Autoimmune Reactivity. This test looks at the brain proteins themselves and assists in early detection of neuroautoimmunity, evaluates severity of the autoimmune response, and helps monitor the effectiveness of treatment protocols. It is recommended for those who show brain function decline with accompanying fatigue or fibromyalgia. This test also checks for gluten reactivity and dairy sensitivity contributing to neurological dysfunction. (Cyrex Laboratories)

Array 8: Joint Autoimmune Reactivity Screen. This panel looks at the joint tissue itself and tests for immunoglobulin G and immunoglobulin A antibodies. It is recommended for those with arthritis, arthralgias, or joint inflammation following exposure to environmental triggers. It's also helpful in early detection of connective tissue disorders and monitoring the effectiveness of treatment protocols. (Cyrex Laboratories)

Array 10: Multiple Food Immune Reactivity Screen. This panel provides early detection of food-related reactivity and evaluates reactions to raw and cooked foods, food enzymes, lectins, and artificial food additives, including meat glue, colorings, and gums. It's recommended for those who suspect increased intestinal permeability and those with unexplained symptoms, whether gastrointestinal, neurological, dermatological, or behavioral in nature. (Cyrex Laboratories)

Array 20: Blood–Brain Barrier Permeability Screen. This is for those experiencing brain fog, memory loss, or a history of prior head trauma. Since leaky gut can be connected to leaky brain (covered in Chapter 6), this test screens for serum antibodies to the protein structures that constitute the blood-brain barrier. It is recommended for those who show abnormal elevations in lipopolysaccharides or occludin and zonulin antibody levels. It's often performed in tandem with the Array 2: Intestinal Antigenic Permeability Screen. (Cyrex Laboratories)

ELISA tests for antibodies in the blood and is the gold standard for identifying food immune reactivity. In the

MY TEST RESULTS CAME BACK NORMAL—BUT I DON'T FEEL NORMAL

Physicians are often faced with patients who have a history of unexplained, non-specific, chronic symptoms. These often include fatigue, malaise, muscle and joint aches, low-grade fevers, irritable bowel symptoms, sleep disturbance, mental fogginess, blurred vision, unusual headaches, dizzy spells, short-term memory loss, and cognitive function problems. Typically, these patients have previously sought help from other doctors, who ran the usual tests with mostly normal findings. Despite the results, the patients' symptoms continue.

Normal readings are common in patients with food immune reactivities. So-called "normal" reference ranges in standard laboratory testing are based on a control group of healthy people. The range helps show what a typical result looks like, but it doesn't explain everything for everyone. Some healthy people test outside the range and some unhealthy people test within it. If you still have symptoms despite normal results, you likely need additional testing.

NOTES FROM THE LAB

Steroids and immunosuppressant drugs can interfere with the results of immunological tests, so be sure to talk to your health care practitioner about potentially pausing them three weeks before testing. For fecal tests, avoid red meat, vitamin C-rich foods and beverages, pain relievers such as aspirin and ibuprofen, and certain fruits and vegetables like beets, broccoli, and turnips. Ask your health care expert about other drugs, foods, or supplements you may need to pause or stop taking.

Many doctors, including me, prefer to test patients in their usual state, especially if that includes medications. In some situations, such as preparing for a skin prick test, you should avoid antihistamines, vitamin C, vitamin A, CoQ10, and gingko biloba in the five days leading up to the test.

Food immune reactivity testing involves checking for immunoglobulin G. If you suspect sensitivity (but not a severe reaction) to a particular food, such as wheat, consume some in the month prior to testing to ensure antibodies are still circulating through your system. Otherwise, you may receive a false negative.

lab, blood samples are placed in miniature test tubes and exposed to a variety of food antigens. If the blood contains antibodies to the antigen, the two will bind together. (Cyrex Laboratories)

Thyroid Peroxidase and Thyroglobulin Test is a simple blood test that looks for autoantibodies targeting the thyroid. These develop when a person's immune system mistakenly targets components of the thyroid gland or thyroid proteins, leading to chronic inflammation of the thyroid (thyroiditis), tissue damage, and disruption of thyroid function. (Labcorp or Quest Diagnostics)

GAM Total Serum Immunoglobulins assesses overall production of IgG, IgA, and IgM antibodies—an important measurement of general immunity. Total immunoglobulins testing can be a strong indicator of a disease or condition and is recommended when immunodeficiency is suspected. (Quest Diagnostics, Labcorp, or Cyrex Laboratories)

Immunotype testing (CD4/CD8/CD3/CD19/NK cells count) looks at the makeup of your T cells, B cells, and natural killer cells to determine whether there are imbalances or deficiencies. (Quest Diagnostics, Labcorp, or Cyrex Laboratories)

Complete blood cell count with differential (CBC) is a group of tests that measures the concentration of cells circulating in the bloodstream, including red blood cells (RBCs), white blood cells (WBCs), and platelets (PLTs). The CBC can evaluate your overall health and detect a variety of diseases and conditions, including infections. (Labcorp or Quest Diagnostics)

Antinuclear antibody test (ANA) detects autoantibodies in the blood and can determine whether a patient has an autoimmune disease such as lupus, scleroderma, and rheumatoid arthritis. (Immunosciences Lab, Labcorp, or Quest Diagnostics)

Antineutrophil Cytoplasmic Antibodies (ANCA) are autoantibodies produced when the immune system mistakenly targets its own neutrophil proteins. This test checks for their presence and is often used when inflammation of the blood vessels is suspected. (Labcorp or Quest Diagnostics)

HLA-B27 tests for the presence of human leukocyte antigen B27 (HLA-B27), an indicator that the immune system is attacking its own tissues. (Labcorp or Quest Diagnostics)

GI 360 or CDSA stool test detects and assesses the status of pathogens, viruses, parasites, and bacteria that may be contributing to acute or chronic gastrointestinal symptoms and disease. (Doctor's Data)

Genetic analysis checks for predispositions; histamine pathways; folate and methionine pathways; methylation cycle; serotonin and melatonin pathways; dopamine, norepinephrine, and epinephrine pathways; and more. (StrateGene)

DETECTING TRIGGERS WITH AN ELIMINATION DIET

Because of my background in developing and reading laboratory tests, I'm a huge proponent of predictive testing. It's the fastest, most concise way to find your genetic predispositions and which foods are triggering your immune responses. If finances or other reasons are holding you back from testing, you can still begin the healing journey.

Start with an elimination diet that replaces the most common inflammatory foods with nutrient-dense, anti-inflammatory items. This method is low-cost, immediately actionable, and very likely to be successful for most people. If you go this route, I highly recommend consulting a registered dietician, nutritionist, or qualified functional medicine doctor before designing your own diet protocol, especially if it's a drastic change for you.

It is much more helpful for individuals with a known autoimmune disease to order a full food reactivity panel that includes culprits like gluten grains, dairy, eggs, lectins, and meat, as well as fish, shellfish, spices, nuts, fruit, and aquaporins (corn, spinach, soy, and tomato). Remove any foods you test positive for to minimize inflammation and autoimmune responses.

PRO-INFLAMMATORY FOODS TO ELIMINATE PERMANENTLY

Proteins, including bacon with nitrates, conventionally raised meat, hot dogs, lunch meats, and meat cooked or fried at very high temperatures.

Gluten-containing grains, cereals, and baked goods, including barley, breads, bulgur, cereals, couscous, emmer, farro, freekeh, kamut, some oats, pasta, pastries, rye, spelt, wheat germ, and wheat.

Gluten-containing compounds, including barbecue sauce, binders, bouillon, brewer's yeast, chewing gum, condiments, emulsifiers, fillers, hot dogs, hydrolyzed plant and animal protein, ketchup, lunch meats, malt and malt flavoring, malt vinegar, matzo, modified food starch, monosodium glutamate, non-dairy creamer, processed salad dressings, seitan, some spice mixtures, soy sauce, stabilizers, teriyaki sauce, and texturized vegetable protein.

Most beans and legumes, including peas, peanuts, pinto beans, and soybeans.

High-glycemic alcohol, including beer, dark liquors, hard ciders, and sweet wines.

Sweeteners and drinks such as agave syrup, all energy drinks and sodas (including diet), artificial sweeteners (Equal, Splenda, Sweet'N Low, Truvia, or anything else that contains isomalt, maltitol, mannitol, sorbitol, or xylitol), brown sugar, evaporated cane juice, high-fructose corn syrup, powdered sugar, and white sugar.

Soy products, including edamame, soy milk, soy protein, soy sauce, and tofu. Exceptions are fermented soy products.

Refined oils, including margarine, and seed and vegetable oils like canola, corn, grapeseed, sunflower, safflower, and soybean.

Others, including additives like gums and food coloring, canned foods, and all other heavily processed foods.

POTENTIAL TRIGGER FOODS TO ELIMINATE TEMPORARILY

During the elimination phase, temporarily remove all of the following items from your diet for thirty to sixty days. Depending on the severity of your symptoms, you may need to go longer. If you suspect other foods of wreaking havoc and they're not listed here, remove those too. We'll go over how to reintroduce these items in the next section.

Aquaporins, including corn, spinach, soy, and tomato.

Beans and legumes, including soaked or sprouted lentils, black beans, and chickpeas.

Nightshades, including eggplant, goji berries, peppers, tomatillos, tomatoes, and white potatoes.
Non-gluten grain and flours, including amaranth, buckwheat, quinoa, rice, sorghum, millet, cassava, and teff.

Dairy products, eggs, and egg-based condiments, including aioli, béarnaise, butter, buttermilk, cheese, chicken eggs, cottage cheese, duck eggs, ghee, Greek yogurt (unsweetened), heavy cream, mayonnaise, sour cream, and whey.

Nuts and seeds, including almonds, Brazil nuts, cashews, chia, cocoa, chocolate, coffee, flaxseeds, hemp seeds, macadamias nuts, nut and seed milks, nut butters, pecans, pistachios, sesame seeds, sunflower seeds, and walnuts.

Fermented soy products, including miso, natto, and tempeh.

Spices, including allspice, anise, cardamom, caraway, celery seed, coriander, cumin, dill seed, fennel seed, juniper, mustard seed, nutmeg, and pepper (black and white).

Natural sweeteners, including coconut sugar, dates, honey, molasses, monk fruit extract, pure maple syrup, raw honey, and Stevia.

Low-glycemic alcohol, including clear liquors and dry wines.

AUTOIMMUNE PROTOCOL FOODS TO ENJOY FOR LIFE

Elimination diets are a great way to heal the gut and turn off the genes that cause autoimmunity. Below is the wonderful array of foods you can consume freely and abundantly, unless otherwise noted.

Grass-fed, hormone-free, nitrate-free, and wild-caught proteins, including beef, bison, chicken, duck, elk, halibut, lamb, liver, lobster, salmon, sardines, scallops, sea bass, squid, tripe, trout, tuna (not canned), and turkey. If you're not allergic to shellfish, you can include clams, crab, mussels, oysters, and shrimp as well. Farm-raised clams, mussels, and oysters are fine.

Organic vegetables, including artichoke, arugula, asparagus, bok choy, broccoli, brussels sprouts, butternut squash, cabbage, cauliflower, celery, chard, chives, cucumber, endive, fennel, kale, leeks, lettuce, mushrooms, okra, onions, plantains, radicchio, radish, rhubarb, shallots, sprouts (especially cruciferous sprouts such as broccoli, radish, kale, and mustard greens), sweet potatoes, water chestnuts, and zucchini.

Low-glycemic fruits, including blueberries, cherries, cranberries, raspberries, and strawberries. Higher glycemic fruits can be consumed in moderation but no more than 10 to 20 grams per day. These include apples, bananas, blackberries, cantaloupe, citrus, figs, grapes, kiwi, mangoes, peaches, pears, pineapples, plums, pomegranate, and watermelon.

Fermented foods, including apple cider vinegar, coconut yogurt or kefir (unsweetened), kimchi, kombucha tea, kvass, pickles, pickled ginger, and sauerkraut.

Beverages, including bone broth, filtered water, sparkling water, and unsweetened teas (caffeinated and herbal).

Herbs and spices, including basil, bay leaf, chive, cilantro, cinnamon, clove, curry, dill (herb), garlic, ginger, horseradish, lemongrass, oregano, parsley, peppermint, rosemary, saffron, sage, spearmint, tarragon, thyme, turmeric, and vanilla extract (gluten-free). Pink Himalayan salt may be used sparingly.

Fats and oils, including avocado oil, avocados, coconut butter, coconut milk (unsweetened), coconut oil, extra-virgin olive oil, lard, MCT oil, and olives.

REINTRODUCING FOODS BACK INTO YOUR DIET

After a couple of weeks on the elimination diet, you should notice a considerable difference in your health, with no bloating, gas, constipation, or diarrhea. You may also notice your thinking is clearer and you feel lighter after a meal.

At this stage, you're ready to gauge your sensitivity to the foods you removed and reintroduce some back into your diet. Start with spices and wait several days. Then move on to eggs and wait a few days. Continue in the same fashion with nuts and seeds, nightshades, dairy, and low-glycemic alcohol last. Use artificial sweeteners in moderation, and continue to avoid foods you reacted to immunologically on a blood test.

If you're symptom-free for several days after reintroducing a food, you can assume your body tolerates it well and introduce another. If, however, you encounter some issues, assume the food does not agree with you. Permanently remove that specific food from your diet and wait a week for the inflammation to clear out of your body before reintroducing another food.

DETECTING TRIGGER FOODS

Know the signs. Your body is a terrific communicator—if you pay careful attention to the messages it sends. Symptoms and common indicators of food immune reactivity to look out for include:

- Acid reflux
- Abdominal pain
- Bloating
- Brain fog
- Digestive issues
- Diarrhea
- Fatigue
- Headaches or migraines
- Irritability
- Joint pain
- Mood changes such as depression or anxiety
- Nausea or vomiting
- Poor sleep or insomnia
- Rashes, hives, or skin irritations
- Sinus issues

Document your journey. It helps to keep a record of your symptoms as you gradually detect which foods you can and cannot tolerate. Pay attention to your patterns and take note in a daily journal when you experience something new or unexpected. Monitor how well you sleep, whether you wake up energized or groggy, any sudden weight loss or gain, changes in mood or bowel habits, and energy drops. Document how you feel after removing a food from your diet and how you feel when you reintroduce it.

Monitor your bowels. Your gut should express itself every day through a bowel movement. Each gut is different, of course, but a healthy one typically follows a consistent pattern. One of the best indicators of gut imbalance or inflammation is the shape, consistency, frequency, and color of your stool, so make sure to glance in the toilet before you flush to check its condition. You may have a gut issue if your bowel movement:

- happens several times a day or not at all
- is runny, loose, or not well formed
- presents as small pebbles, multiple pieces, or clumpy
- is green, black, yellow, or clay colored
- is filled with mucus
- is filled with undigested food (except small seeds like chia, flax, or sunflower)

By comparison, a healthy bowel movement:
- passes swiftly
- happens only once or twice every day
- drops to the bottom of the toilet
- is a consistent variance of brown
- is soft to firm in texture and well formed in one or a few pieces

5

FOLLOW YOUR GUT

Every man is the builder of a temple, called his body.

– Henry David Thoreau

The Western world is currently experiencing an alarming increase in gut inflammatory disorders—from small intestinal bacterial overgrowth and irritable bowel syndrome to Crohn's disease, ulcerative colitis, celiac disease, and non-celiac gluten sensitivity. For answers, we need look no further than the loss of our ancestral microbiome.

Simply put, our guts no longer resemble those of our ancestors. Instead of a microbiome teeming with friendly bacteria working symbiotically with our immune systems, our guts are weakened by modern-day toxins. This almost certainly accounts for the increase in gut dysbiosis, where bad bacteria take over the good, setting us up for inflammation and increased intestinal permeability.

Aggressive immune responses directed to your digestive system can result in common things like bloating and acid reflux. They can also develop into a more complex autoimmune disease. Following are some of the more common types of gut-centered autoimmunity.

Inflammatory bowel disease (IBD) is an umbrella term for a group of individual intestinal diseases, including Crohn's disease, microscopic colitis, and ulcerative colitis. IBD affects the bowel wall, causing inflammation, sores, and narrowing of the intestines. Symptoms can come and go, and include chronic diarrhea, abdominal cramps, anemia, blocked bowels, bloody stool, fever, loss of appetite, and weight loss.

In Crohn's disease, inflammation presents anywhere along the digestive tract, from the mouth and esophagus to the small intestine, appendix, large intestines, and anus. Many people living with Crohn's have compromised immune systems, and it most often strikes in younger populations, ages fifteen to thirty-five. Other symptoms might include abdominal pain on the right side, rashes, anal fissures, and joint pain.

Microscopic colitis is an autoimmune and inflammatory condition of the large intestine, typically causing chronic watery diarrhea. Though this condition used to be considered rare, new data suggest its prevalence is growing rapidly. Currently, it can be detected only through colonoscopy with an intestinal

CASE STUDY: BRAD

Brad, a thirty-six-year-old man, lived a stereotypical bachelor life. A social drinker who preferred takeout over home-cooked meals, he had a casual workout regimen, ate a lot of bread, and sometimes splurged by stocking his pantry with sugary breakfast pastries. He came to me with concerns about his debilitating abdominal pain, bloating, and two to three runny stools a day. To further intensify his condition, he had cyclical episodes of severe diarrhea and cramping every three months. He also suffered from seasonal allergies and took an antihistamine daily.

Prior to our meeting, Brad had seen three gastrointestinal doctors before a fourth diagnosed him with irritable bowel syndrome, or IBS. He had been prescribed high-dose probiotics and an antibiotic called rifaximin, commonly used in IBS patients because it isn't absorbed into the bloodstream and stays in the gut. Despite temporary relief, Brad's loose stools returned and his doctor put him on several more rounds of the antibiotic, to no avail.

Detect the problem: Due to the longevity of Brad's condition and his repeated antibiotic use, we tested him for general food reactivity, leaky gut, and non-celiac gluten sensitivity. He had previously tested negative on celiac tests, so I wanted to rule out gluten entirely with the precise testing that Cyrex Arrays 2 and 3X provide. As suspected, his test came back positive for severe leaky gut and non-celiac gluten sensitivity. This meant that gluten was the trigger for his GI autoimmune response, and prolonged consumption had broken down his oral tolerance. The cascading inflammation led to a leaky gut. Had we not caught this, the inflammation might have eventually reached other organs in his body, causing disease in the brain, skin, and joints.

Remove the triggers: Brad immediately restricted all gluten from his diet.

Repair the barrier: Brad's regimen included daily supplements of high-dose probiotics (100 billion CFUs), oral glutathione, glutamine, and turmeric to repair the inflammatory damage caused by antibiotics and gluten, restore his microbiome, and revitalize his leaky system.

Results: Four weeks later, Brad's abdominal pain, bloating, and diarrhea had completely resolved. As an added bonus, his seasonal allergies had significantly improved too. In the months that followed, Brad reported that he was sleeping better, felt less puffy, and felt less joint pain, and his daily bowel movements had normalized. By this stage, he had been anticipating his quarterly episode of severe pain and diarrhea, but it never came. Six months into treatment, all of Brad's symptoms had disappeared.

---

biopsy, but researchers are working toward a blood test. Besides diarrhea, common symptoms include abdominal pain, cramping, fecal incontinence, and weight loss. Contributing factors include leaky gut, food allergies, food immune reactivity, and chronic use of NSAIDs such as aspirin or ibuprofen.

Another factor is the presence of yeast or "bad" bacteria in the gut that can produce endotoxins like lipopolysaccharides or exotoxins such as bacterial cytolethal distending toxin found in *salmonella, Shigella,* and *Campylobacter jejuni.* (An exotoxin is secreted by bacteria outside the cell, while endotoxins are bacterial toxins located within a cell. When the cell disintegrates, the endotoxin is released.)

In ulcerative colitis, the cells in the lining of the large intestine die off and create open ulcers, often causing pus, mucus, and bleeding. Symptoms include bloody diarrhea, chronic fatigue, loss of appetite, malnutrition, and anemia, along with joint pain, kidney stones, rashes, osteoporosis, and liver disorders. Like Crohn's, ulcerative colitis often begins at a young age but is also seen in the elderly.

Despite its similar name and acronym, irritable bowel syndrome (IBS) differs from IBD. Rather than affecting the intestinal wall, IBS affects bowel function. But like IBD, it can affect both the small and large intestines and present similar symptoms, including gassiness, abdominal pain, bloating (especially after carbohydrate consumption), diarrhea or constipation (or a combination of both), and incomplete defecation. IBS often overlaps with other disorders, including chronic fatigue, small intestinal bacterial overgrowth (SIBO), migraine headaches, scleroderma, celiac disease, and more.

A physician might treat each of these issues individually without realizing they're all connected. On the other end of the treatment spectrum, a patient might receive a blanket diagnosis when they're in need of specialized treatment. For example, one person might need to eliminate gluten and dairy. For another, it could mean removing eggs or red food dye. Someone else might need antibiotics for a bacterial infection. Yet all are treated similarly, often with antibiotics, under the false assumption they have an infection.

When diagnosing IBS, doctors consider the patient's medical history, which might include unintentional weight loss, anemia, recurrent nausea and vomiting, as well as a family history of inflammatory bowel disease. Immunoglobulin G antibodies against food antigens for wheat, milk, eggs, and corn are often found in inflammatory bowel diseases.

Astonishingly, 15 percent of all patient visits to primary care physicians and 25 to 50 percent of all visits to gastrointestinal specialists are for conditions related to IBS. It is the most common gastrointestinal disorder in the United States, but up to 75 percent of those living with the syndrome will go undiagnosed for years. Factors that can contribute to IBS include genetics, stress, toxin exposure, leaky gut, and dysbiosis.

Small intestinal bacterial overgrowth (SIBO) often occurs alongside IBS. Up to 84 percent of IBS patients also live with SIBO, which develops when bacteria from the colon backs up into the small intestine and begins to cultivate. When this happens, homeostasis, or balance, in the GI tract is lost and necessary digestive enzymes and nutrients such as B12 and iron are depleted. People with SIBO can experience unexplained weight loss, malnutrition, and possibly osteoporosis.

In both IBS and SIBO, contributing factors include an overworked immune system, an overgrowth of bacteria, molecular mimicry, food antigens, and leaky gut. When the immune system shifts into overdrive, it can affect the balance of good bacteria in your gut, resulting in an overgrowth of bacterial toxins such as *E. coli* and *salmonella*. The bacterial endotoxin called lipopolysaccharide is also released.

Because the structures of *E. coli* and *salmonella* (as well as *Shigella*, which causes dysentery, and *Campylobacter jejuni*, which causes bacterial food poisoning) are similar to the proteins found in the gut lining, molecular mimicry can also enter the picture.

NOTES FROM THE LAB

People with irritable bowel syndrome sometimes swear off cruciferous vegetables like broccoli, cauliflower, brussels sprouts, and cabbage, since the dietary sulfur they contain can cause uncomfortable gas and bloating. However, these vegetables actually help heal the gut, because they contain a distinct chemical compound called indole-3-carbinol that helps regulate mucosal immune function.

For sensitive bellies, I recommend introducing these veggies in the form of young sprouts and leaves. For instance, broccoli and radish sprouts contain all the powerful healing properties without the hard-to-digest fiber. Leafy greens in this category include arugula, bok choy, collard greens, mustard greens, kale, swiss chard, and watercress, and work well in salads or stir-fries. Start light with the sprouts and gradually build up to small servings of the leafy varieties to find your level of tolerance. Over time, you may be able to increase the size of your servings as you progress on your healing journey.

KNOW THE SIGNS
When autoimmunity attacks the digestive tract, you may experience:
- A distended stomach
- A feeling of tightness around the belly
- Brain fog the day after eating a trigger food
- Gassiness or bloating

Common Trigger Foods in This Category
- Corn
- Cereal grains
- Dairy
- Eggs
- Gluten
- Lectins (legumes and nightshades)
- Soy

Risk Factors
- An altered microbiome either from birth via C-section or early antibiotic use
- Anatomic alterations (such as leaky gut or gastric bypass surgery)
- Exposure to chemicals
- Failure of either the gastric acid barrier or small intestinal motility
- Food allergies and intolerances
- Loss of oral tolerance
- Medications such as antibiotics or NSAIDs
- Overconsumption of sugar, processed foods, and toxic additives

Recommended Tests
- Array 2: Intestinal Antigenic Permeability Screen (Cyrex Laboratories)
- Food sensitivity testing, as appropriate

If I suspect cross-reactivity with gluten, I'll include:
- Array 4: Gluten-Associated Cross-Reactive Foods and Foods Sensitivity (Cyrex Laboratories)

For a full food reactivity screen, I'll order:
- Array 10: Multiple Food Immune Reactivity Screen (Cyrex Laboratories)

Remember, zonulin and occludin are proteins responsible for opening tight junctions. If you test positive for immunoglobulin G and immunoglobulin A autoantibodies against these proteins, it indicates a problem with leaky gut. If you test positive for an antibody called actomyosin, a protein found in muscle tissue, it signals a breakdown of the intestinal wall. The presence of lipopolysaccharides antibodies indicates dysbiosis, or the overgrowth of harmful bacteria in relation to good.

Celiac disease (CD) is an immune reaction to gluten that affects an estimated 3 million Americans. In the last decade, the numbers have increased threefold. When people with celiac eat gluten, they typically have an immediate gut-centered inflammatory reaction like severe bloating, diarrhea, fatigue, brain fog, depression, anxiety, migraines, joint pain, and more. By comparison, people with non-celiac gluten sensitivity (NCGS) experience similar symptoms when they consume gluten yet test negative for celiac.

The main difference between the two is celiac has a genetic component, while non-celiac gluten sensitivity is linked to the activation of the innate immune system. It is detected by a blood test that looks for IgG and IgA antibodies to gluten peptides and the absence of antibodies to tissue transglutaminases (a test patented by my father).

Patients with a confirmed diagnosis for celiac disease are prescribed a gluten-free diet and improve significantly in a six-month time span. Meanwhile, non-celiac gluten sensitivity patients continue eating gluten because their tests came back negative.

Over time, the inflammation in their guts is compounded, potentially leading to gut dysbiosis, neuroinflammation, gut-brain axis dysfunction, and vulnerability to other autoimmune disorders. In most cases, medications are prescribed to mask these symptoms. Unfortunately, these medications eventually stop working because the root cause of the illness is not being accurately identified and treated.

Both conditions appear to play a significant role in endocrine disorders, reported in 4 to 8 percent of women with unexplained infertility. Today, 13 million Americans are living with non-celiac gluten sensitivity.

6

THE BRAIN AND NERVOUS SYSTEM

We are designed to be smart people our entire lives.
The brain is supposed to work well until our last breath.

– David Perlmutter, MD

The brain is an amazingly complex organ. Weighing in at around three pounds, it contains 100 billion neurons and over 400 miles of blood vessels, mostly capillaries. Your gut and brain share similar characteristics, including identical capillaries that are vastly different from the other 10 billion or so that traverse your body.

These highly specialized capillaries make up your blood-brain barrier (BBB), which also connect to the capillaries in your intestinal barrier. Like the protective lining of your gut, your blood-brain barrier is lined with an extensive network of endothelial cells and tight junctions designed to be highly selective.

Like the gatekeeper it is, the blood-brain barrier allows the passage of essential metabolites and lipid soluble molecules such as oxygen, carbon dioxide, hormones, and glucose while simultaneously blocking access to toxins, infections, and the byproducts of infection like lipopolysaccharides (LPS). In sum, your blood-brain barrier, when working properly, helps you to maintain cerebral homeostasis.

Unfortunately, if your gut is leaky, chances are your brain is too, as the two are closely linked in a symbiotic relationship known as the gut-brain axis. The large vagus nerve runs between the brain and the digestive system, relaying communication back and forth. When your gut is leaky, bacteria, yeast, toxins, and large molecules of undigested food proteins gain entry into the circulatory system. Over time, these pathogens eventually gain entry through the blood-brain barrier, potentially causing neuroinflammation, neurodegeneration, and neuroautoimmunity.

The gut also has its own nervous system—called the enteric nervous system (ENS)—composed of the same kind of nerve cells and neurochemicals found in the brain. If you've ever had the feeling of butterflies fluttering around inside you or felt knots in your stomach, you've experienced crosstalk between your gut and brain. This sophisticated means of communication has been going on since birth and plays a significant role in how your brain is hardwired. It can even influence your mood.

CASE STUDY: MEGAN

Megan, a thirty-six-year-old woman, presented with frequent migraines. They were so debilitating, in fact, that she was forced to call in sick to work, often for several days at a time. She also experienced eczema, chronic sinusitis, and seasonal allergies. Her life was driven by these crippling recurrences and the never-ending inconvenience of allergies.

Several ear, nose, and throat doctors blamed allergies for the migraines, but they never pinpointed the cause for the constant sneezing, sniffling, and itching. Consequently, Megan relied on an antihistamine during the day and a stronger antihistamine at night, and a steroid nasal spray when she needed additional relief. At least once a year, she experienced a nasty sinus infection that required antibiotics. Still, Megan's migraines persisted, which necessitated prescription and over-the-counter pain relievers.

Despite the constant flow of medications, Megan's migraines and chronic sinus infections continued. This was the condition she was in when she sat down with me to discuss her set of prolonged, disabling symptoms.

Detect the problem: We dug deep into Megan's lifestyle, medical history, exposure to pollutants, and dietary habits. She ate clean but with regular gluten and dairy indulgences. When I asked her about bowel movements, she revealed that she passed one hard, small stool every other day. Assuming this was normal, she was shocked when I explained that a normal bowel movement should happen daily and resembles not a pebble but a snake, soft to firm in texture and passed painlessly, without strain.

Due to Megan's gastrointestinal issues, I ordered the Array 2: Intestinal Antigenic Permeability Screen to confirm leaky gut, along with other tests to detect any food intolerances. The results showed elevated antibodies to gluten peptides, dairy, and buckwheat. The permeability screen also revealed unusually high antibodies to actomyosin, a complex set of proteins found in muscle fibers. Actomyosin is also found throughout the muscular lining of the small intestine, so when antibodies for it show up in the bloodstream, it's a pretty clear indicator of intestinal damage and increased permeability.

Remove the triggers: Megan immediately eliminated gluten, dairy, and buckwheat from her diet.

Repair the barrier: To reduce inflammation and rebuild the gut lining, I prescribed a daily serving of collagen-rich bone broth. I also gave her bromelain (pineapple extract), vitamin C, and a spore-based probiotic called MegaSporeBiotic. For most people, healing generally takes place over three months, but we aimed for six months in Megan's case since her immune functions and intestinal lining were severely impaired.

Results: Three months later, in the dead of winter when Megan's symptoms historically were exacerbated, she didn't need to take her annual dose of antibiotics. Her constipation was replaced with well-formed daily bowel movements, and her chronic sinus infection and runny nose were 75 percent better. She reported that she was sleeping better, had more energy, and felt mentally sharper. By the six-month mark, all of Megan's symptoms had vanished, and she was migraine-free for the first time in fifteen years. Though I'm highlighting a clinical success story here, it's important to mention that not all outcomes are this good. The earlier these efforts and changes are made for an individual in the course of their disease, the more likely they are to succeed.

Thoughts, stress, and traumatic events trigger chemical reactions inside your brain, which you then experience as an emotion. These chemical responses send a variety of reactions throughout your body, most intensely to your gut. This is why emotions like anger, anxiety, or sadness are often felt there.

The gut-brain connection also promotes proper digestion and plays a role in intuition, which explains "gut feelings" and "gut instincts." The link between the two is so powerful that the gut is often dubbed the "second brain." The communication goes both ways, so when there is inflammation or degeneration in the gut, it can manifest as depression, anxiety, irritability, brain fog, or migraines.

Not only can your gut health alter your mood but it can also affect your very personality. For example, a study on mice showed that the composition of gut bacteria can cause mice to be either timid and shy or boisterous and adventurous. Scientists were able to make the timid mice bolder and more adventurous simply by killing their gut bacteria with antibiotics and then inoculating their guts with bacteria from the bolder mice and the reverse.

Gut bacteria influence human behavior as well. For instance, chronic gut inflammation has been shown to cause chronic anxiety, and the presence of the endotoxin lipopolysaccharides in the bloodstream is linked with major depression. We also now know that around 35 percent of people living with depression have leaky gut. The good news is that people with neurological health issues often show a measurable improvement after receiving probiotics.

COMMON GUT-BRAIN AUTOIMMUNE DISORDERS

According to the Centers for Disease Control and Prevention (CDC), cognitive impairment now affects 16 million Americans. Sadly, data projections show that this number will double within the next twenty years. Today more than 40 million Americans are living with preclinical dementia, meaning they're heading toward mental decline. One of the biggest health threats we currently face is neuroautoimmunity. This section covers some of the brain disorders affected by food immune reactivity and reveals how GI inflammation can make its way up to the brain.

Alzheimer's disease is the most common form of dementia, contributing up to 70 percent of all cases and currently affecting 44 million people worldwide. In the U.S., one person in every five over age sixty-five has mild cognitive impairment, and one in seven has been diagnosed with dementia. As staggering as these statistics are, they're expected to triple by 2050.

In Alzheimer's, deposits of beta-amyloid proteins build up in neural tissue and cause brain cells degenerate. Normally, beta-amyloids aren't harmful to the body and play an essential role in neural growth and repair. As we age, corrupted beta-amyloids can accumulate and form plaques that block communication between cells.

It was once thought (and still is for some) that Alzheimer's was purely genetic, but that is not the case. In recent years, researchers have turned to the effects of a diet high in processed carbohydrates and an unhealthy gut microbiome. In fact, many are looking more closely at the link between harmful gut bacteria—like E. coli and salmonella—and the rise of poor brain health.

NOTES FROM THE LAB
Most middle-age people are familiar with the idea of getting colonoscopies by age fifty to check for precancerous lesions that can develop into something more serious. As Dale E. Bredesen, MD, author of The End of Alzheimer's, suggests, we need to do something similar for our brains. He writes, "The way for all of us over forty-five years old to prevent cognitive decline is to have a 'cognoscopy,' evaluating all of the potential contributors and risk factors." I wholeheartedly agree. Predictive testing can detect potential issues years in advance and give you the opportunity to remove triggers from your environment and prevent neuroautoimmunity from taking hold.

CASE STUDY: PAUL

Paul, a forty-five-year-old man, came to me with a history of debilitating fatigue that left him bedridden most days. His brain fog was so severe that pulling together a simple thought felt like dragging a truck out of the mud. Because his exhaustion and brain fog began to mirror the signs of depression, he had visited a psychiatrist. When antidepressants failed to address Paul's symptoms, his psychiatrist referred him to me, with the understanding that chronic fatigue and brain fog are often the result of poor diet rather than emotional despair.

Detect the problem: During our consultation, Paul didn't initially realize he had intestinal issues, because he didn't exhibit any loud alarms like diarrhea or constipation. He did, however, experience bloating with abdominal distension after eating. Unfortunately, quiet alarms like this often go unnoticed or get dismissed even though they often prove critical in detecting an underlying condition. We tested Paul for leaky gut, which came back positive with the presence of lipopolysaccharides in the bloodstream, the hallmark of a condition known as chronic endotoxemia, which is known to cause significant neuroinflammation and brain fog. Paul's tests also revealed food immune reactivity to gluten and soy.

Remove the triggers: Paul eliminated gluten and soy from his diet.

Repair the barrier: We added daily supplements including oral glutamine, vitamin D3, and the probiotic MegaSporeBiotic to repair his gut damage.

Results: Three months later, Paul's brain fog was completely resolved. He reported sleeping well through the night and waking up with sustained energy throughout the day.

Some of the top contributing factors include prior infections, hormone imbalances, toxic exposure to things like heavy metals or mold, and head injuries, along with diet, food immune reactivity, and gut disorders such as irritable bowel syndrome, or IBS.

To determine the foods that exacerbate the buildup of beta-amyloid, my father and I checked for cross-reactivity between beta-amyloid peptides and a variety of food antigens. The food antigens that reacted most strongly were wheat proteins (both gluten and non-gluten) and milk caseins.

In one experiment, we took a random blood sampling of 400 supposedly healthy people. The results showed that 20 percent reacted to gluten and casein, and 50 percent of those people demonstrated autoimmunity to brain tissue—meaning autoimmunity was silently unfolding without their knowledge. Left untreated, early symptoms have the potential to progress into any number of different autoimmune disorders, including multiple sclerosis, Alzheimer's, Parkinson's, balance issues, mood disorders, migraines, depression, and so on.

The gut also relates to Alzheimer's. The bacteria that live in the digestive tract produce beta-amyloids and lipopolysaccharides (the byproduct of infection). When the gates of the gut open and beta-amyloids and lipopolysaccharides make their way into the circulatory system, they produce inflammatory cytokines. Increased proinflammatory cytokine secretion then contributes to the onset of insulin resistance, a recognized risk factor for Alzheimer's.

But there is good news in all of this. We now know that about twenty years before the telltale signs of Alzheimer's appear, patients experience a clinical phase where changes are going on inside the brain but no symptoms are present. This powerful knowledge provides us with much hope, because through predictive testing we can now detect this disease many, many years in advance before the damage sets in. This gives us an opportunity to fix the problem at its root cause before the disease can take hold.

Attention deficit/hyperactivity disorder (ADHD) is an umbrella term for three subtypes of brain-based syndromes: inattentive (traditionally called attention deficit disorder, or ADD), hyperactive-impulse (ADHD), and a combination of the two. The disorders affect attention, concentration, memory, motivation and effort, learning from mistakes, impulsivity, hyperactivity, organization, and social skills. According to epidemiological data, 11 million Americans have ADHD, including 5 percent of the adult population. Genetics is often considered the number one factor contributing to ADHD, but chemical influences can also play a part.

For example, synthetic food coloring found in cereals, cupcakes, and candies marketed to children can bind to proteins in the body, activating an inflammatory cascade that can ultimately lead to neurobehavioral disorders.

Chronic inflammatory demyelinating polyneuropathy (CIDP) affects the peripheral nerves, causing destruction of the nerves' fatty protective covering, called myelin. Myelin allows the nerves to transmit signals, but when it's damaged, it gradually produces weakness associated with loss of reflexes. Affecting about one or two people per 100,000, this disease can start at any age and be present in a person for years prior to diagnosis. Unlike most other autoimmune disorders, it's seen more frequently in men than women. Left untreated, 30 percent of CIDP patients will become wheelchair-dependent. Treatment typically involves steroid and plasma exchange, where blood is withdrawn, filtered to remove harmful antibodies, and returned to the body.

Guillain-Barré syndrome (GBS) is an inflammatory disorder targeting the peripheral nerves outside the brain and spinal cord. Symptoms include muscle weakness and tingling and numbness in hands and feet that gradually move to the arms and legs. Sometimes paralysis occurs and can affect breathing muscles. The syndrome affects about one person in 1,000, and roughly two-thirds of people with GBS experience diarrhea or a respiratory illness several weeks before developing symptoms. One of the most common risk factors is an infection with *Campylobacter jejuni*, the bacteria responsible for food poisoning. People can also develop GBS after the flu or other viruses such as cytomegalovirus, Epstein-Barr, and Zika. Treatment sometimes involves a plasma exchange.

Multiple sclerosis (MS) is a severe demyelinating neurological disease. Demyelination happens when the fatty myelin sheaths that surround nerve cells are damaged by inflammation. Damaged myelin impacts the entire body, resulting in cognitive impairment and an onslaught of other symptoms such as fatigue, vertigo, vision problems, numbness, tremor, loss of coordination, depression, and bladder dysfunction. Like most neuroautoimmune disorders, MS is believed to be an inflammatory disorder in which environmental factors, particularly diet, play a significant role.

Backed by a series of global studies, we know that milk is strongly associated with MS. In fact, my father and I found antibodies produced against milk proteins share structural similarities to the human neural tissues myelin basic protein (MBP) and myelin oligodendrocyte glycoprotein (MOG), which could lead to molecular mimicry.

Neuromyelitis optica (NMO), also known as Devic's disease, is an autoimmune disorder similar to MS. With NMO, white blood cells and antibodies primarily attack the optic nerves and the spinal cord but may also attack the brain. The damage to the optic nerves produces swelling and inflammation that cause pain and loss of vision. The damage to the spinal cord causes weakness or paralysis in the legs or arms, loss of sensation, and problems with bladder and bowel function.

NMO is a relapsing-remitting disease. During a relapse, new damage to the optic nerves or spinal cord can lead to accumulating disability. Unlike MS, however, there is no progressive phase to this disease. Consequently, preventing attacks is critical to a good long-term outcome. Again, one of the main causes driving NMO is diet. We know foods like wheat, dairy, and even healthy foods like spinach, corn, tomatoes, and soybeans can play a role in the development of NMO and other neuroautoimmune disorders. We'll discuss these more in Part III of this book, Remove the Triggers.

KNOW THE SIGNS

When autoimmunity attacks the brain and nervous system, you may experience:

- Anxiety
- Attention deficient disorder (ADD)
- Attention deficit/hyperactivity disorder (ADHD)
- Brain fog
- Depression
- Insomnia
- Memory loss
- Migraines
- Obsessive-compulsive disorder (OCD)

Common Trigger Foods in This Category

- Corn
- Dairy
- Eggs
- Gluten
- Soy
- Spinach
- Tomatoes
- Wheat

Recommended Tests

- Array 2: Intestinal Antigenic Permeability Screen (Cyrex Laboratories)
- Array 3X: Wheat/Gluten Proteome Reactivity and Autoimmunity (Cyrex Laboratories)
- Array 4: Gluten-Associated Cross-Reactive Foods and Foods Sensitivity (Cyrex Laboratories)
- Array 7: Neurological Autoimmune Reactivity (Cyrex Laboratories)
- Array 20: Blood–Brain Barrier Permeability Screen (Cyrex Laboratories)

Obsessive-compulsive disorder (OCD) is recognized for repetitive behavior and intrusive thoughts that can interfere with daily life. Many people exhibit some degree of obsessive or compulsive tendencies, but in clinical terms, it's the need to perform a specific function, such as repeatedly washing hands, locking and unlocking doors, and compulsive cleaning. If a person with OCD is unable to carry out the action repeatedly, anxiety results.

In 1998, the U.S. National Institute of Mental Health identified a subset of OCD called PANDAS (Pediatric Autoimmune Neuropsychiatric Disorders Associated with Streptococcal Infections). PANDAS is a neuroinflammatory condition that typically strikes in childhood or early adolescence and occurs when strep infection triggers a misdirected immune response and results in inflammation of the brain. The child quickly begins to exhibit symptoms such as OCD, anxiety, and tics, personality changes such as rage, a decline in math and handwriting abilities, sensory sensitivities, restrictive eating, and more.

PANS (Pediatric Acute-onset Neuropsychiatric Syndrome) was identified more than a decade after PANDAS. The research is still in its infancy, but the triggers include bacterial infections and food reactivity. Though the triggers differ, PANS results in the same hyperactive neuroinflammatory response and life-changing symptoms as PANDAS. In fact, my father wrote a peer-reviewed article in 2020 on this very topic, showing how food reactivity can trigger PANS. He writes that cross-reactivity to a trigger food can bind to neurotransmitter receptors, mimicking an actual neurotransmitter release. Conventional psychiatrists are just starting to understand this neurological disorder, as the science is still emerging, but based on what we know so far, the evidence shows that PANDAS and PANS are both very clearly autoimmune in nature, and like many other autoimmune disorders, involve a dietary component.

Parkinson's disease (PD) is a chronic, progressive disorder typically causing tremor, stiffness, and problems with voluntary movement. One of the better known cases of PD is that of Michael J. Fox, who was diagnosed in 1991 at age twenty-nine. His advocacy and public acknowledgement of his journey have garnered awareness, multitudes of studies, and trials that have led to better understanding of its causes and relief from its symptoms. According to the Michael J. Fox Foundation for Parkinson's Research, between 600,000 and 1 million Americans are living with PD, making it the second most common brain disease after Alzheimer's.

With this disease, neuronal cells in the brain progressively break down and die. These neurons produce dopamine in the region of the brain called the substantia nigra. Dopamine helps the body control movement and coordination, and stimulates feelings of pleasure and reward. As dopamine is lost, symptoms start to develop, including tremors, slowness, balancing issues, and stiffness. For this reason, it is known as a "movement disorder," though memory loss and depression are also common.

Like so many other autoimmune disorders, research initially pointed to genetics as the primary driver. We now know that environmental influences must flip on the genetic switch. Even in the absence of genetic factors, environmental triggers alone can still cause Parkinson's. Some of the triggers include toxic chemicals like pesticides and herbicides, exposure to certain metals like mercury, and head trauma.

Oxidative stress is another contributing factor. This is an imbalance between free radicals and antioxidants, resulting in the formation of neurons called Lewy bodies—the pathological hallmark of Parkinson's disease. Lewy bodies are abnormal clusters of protein that develop inside nerve cells, and their discovery in the intestinal enteric nerves has led to the hypothesis that the first evidence of Parkinson's might actually reside in the GI tract.

Sure enough, many people living with Parkinson's experience bowel problems like constipation. This is in keeping with past studies that found Lewy bodies in the intestinal biopsies of Parkinson's patients. These findings further support the idea that toxins or pathogens travel from the gut to the brain via the enteric nervous system. Once they arrive at a compromised blood-brain barrier, neuroinflammation begins and the progression of Parkinson's unfolds over a period of many years.

WHAT TESTING TELLS US

The intestinal barrier and the blood-brain barrier share similar tight junctions composed of the proteins zonulin, occludin, and claudin, and junctional adhesion molecules (JAM). When we see these markers on a lab test, we can make an educated guess that the blood-brain barrier is compromised along with the intestinal barrier.

Another marker we look for is a byproduct of infection called lipopolysaccharides. In the brain, lipopolysaccharides is linked to major depression and is responsible for opening the tight junctions in the blood-brain barrier. When it escapes into the brain, it can trigger neuroautoimmunity and accelerate brain degeneration. As noted in Chapter 2, T-helper cells 1 and 17 each play a protective role—but when they are overactivated and penetrate the blood-brain barrier, they attack neurons. So we look for the presence of these T-helper cells as well.

Three proteins in the brain also play key roles in the development of neuroautoimmunity: amyloid-beta peptide, alpha-synuclein, and phosphorylated tau. When antibodies against these proteins are produced, they can lead to Alzheimer's and Parkinson's.

7

THE THYROID

Today's opportunities erase yesterday's failures.

– Gene Brown, author

The thyroid is a butterfly-shaped endocrine gland that sits just above the clavicle at the base of your neck. It acts as the body's thermostat, and its job is to help regulate hormones, metabolism, and heart rate. Though small in size—no bigger than a walnut—the thyroid plays a mighty role. It has a tremendous impact on your overall health and well-being, affecting growth, hunger, energy, temperature, muscle control, bone maintenance, brain development, digestive and heart function, and more. When something goes awry inside your body, the thyroid will often be among the first to show signs of poor function.

As part of the endocrine system, your thyroid produces and secretes three types of hormones directly into your bloodstream. The term "thyroid hormone" (TH) generally refers to T4 (thyroxine) and T3 (triiodothyronine) collectively. Too much thyroid hormone and you risk developing Graves' disease; too little and you can end up with Hashimoto's thyroiditis. (The third, calcitonin, helps regulate levels of calcium and phosphate in the bloodstream and is involved in bone metabolism.)

Iodine is one of the building blocks for making T4 and T3 (T4 carries four iodine atoms and T3 has three), and they are the only human cells that absorb iodine. Once the hormones are secreted into your bloodstream, they come in contact with every cell, tissue, and organ in your body. In your liver and certain tissues of your brain, some T4 lose an atom and are converted into T3. It's a delicate balancing act controlled by a messenger chemical called thyroid-stimulating hormone (TSH).

Made by your pituitary, a pea-size gland located deep inside your brain behind your eyeballs, TSH only binds to receptors on cells in the thyroid. The amount of TSH your pituitary makes depends on how much T4 you have circulating throughout your bloodstream. If it's low, your pituitary will produce more TSH to "tell" your thyroid to crank out more T4. Once your T4 reaches a comfortable level, your pituitary gland shuts off its production of TSH.

Unfortunately, 20 million Americans, mostly women, are living with some form of thyroid disease— and up to 60 percent of those people are unaware of their condition. Some estimates suggest that upwards

CASE STUDY: ASHLEY

Ashley, a twenty-three-year-old woman, came to me with an eight-year history of chronic constipation. She led an active social life filled with weekend dining and cocktails and enjoyed a cold beer with chips and dip while watching football. She also loved pizza and indulged frequently. When the constipation became alarmingly uncomfortable, she refocused her diet and ate oats for breakfast, salads for lunch, and veggie-heavy dinners. Still, she was young and spending time with friends, so she continued to surrender to junk food splurges.

Despite her best efforts, Ashley's constipation continued. She began taking anti-inflammatory vitamins and found some relief, but they eventually became ineffective, and that's when she began the doctor runaround. One doctor didn't seem to know where to direct her, while another focused on her hormones. After a blood panel, Ashley was diagnosed with Hashimoto's and put on thyroid replacements.

Three years after this diagnosis, Ashley came to me to wean off the medication and get to the bottom of her condition.

Detect the problem: We tested Ashley for food sensitivities and found immunoglobulin G and immunoglobulin A antibodies for wheat proteins (including wheat germ agglutinin) and immunoglobulin G antibodies for dairy and corn. Other tests came back positive for leaky gut and non-celiac gluten sensitivity. All of Ashley's health issues, including her Hashimoto's, started in the gut, which was reacting to her particular food triggers.

Remove the triggers: Ashley immediately eliminated her dietary triggers with a little help from understanding friends, and said goodbye to pizza, beer, chips, and dip.

Repair the barrier: To help restore Ashley's leaky gut, I put her on probiotics and a supplement called RepairVite (by Apex Energetics).

Results: A month later, Ashley's constipation was nearly resolved, and her abdominal pain was gone. Once she eliminated her specific triggers and healed her leaky gut, her body returned to normal functioning and her hormonal balance was restored. Even better, she was able to go off her thyroid medication, although that isn't possible for all cases.

CASE STUDY: SAMANTHA

Samantha, a thirty-four-year-old woman, came to me with a diagnosis of Hashimoto's and a childhood history of recurrent tonsillitis and sinus infections that were treated with numerous antibiotics in her preteen years. She had typical Hashimoto's symptoms—cold limbs, weight gain, and fatigue—and took 50 micrograms daily of Synthroid, the number one prescribed thyroid medication. Samantha's condition persisted for years despite the medication, so she was eager to manage her condition without it.

Detect the problem: I first tested Samantha's thyroid peroxidase (TPO), which showed extremely high levels at 574. A normal range is less than 30, so this was staggering. Because of her prolonged use of antibiotics, I suspected her gut's microbiome had become greatly impaired, so I wanted to test for leaky gut. There is a medical link between Hashimoto's and leaky gut, so even though she didn't mention intestinal issues, I still wanted to test for it along with food reactivity. Her leaky gut test came back negative, but she showed strong reactivity to wheat peptides and corn, meaning she had circulating antibodies from her triggering food proteins.

Remove the triggers: Samantha embarked on a gluten- and corn-restricted diet, as prescribed.

Repair the barrier: She began a high dose of traditional lacto-bifido probiotics (100 billion CFU) to rebuild her gut flora and maintain general immune balance. I also gave her 5,000 units of vitamin D3, methylated B-complex, and 500 milligrams of curcumin phytosome, the anti-inflammatory component in turmeric.

Results: After one month, Samantha's energy and cold sensation improved. Her TPO labs had dropped from 574 to 300 by month two, leading to a complete resolution in the coldness in her hands and feet. We tapered her Synthroid to half the dose, and at the four-month mark, her TPO antibodies were 78, her thyroid hormones were within normal range, and we removed Synthroid completely from her daily regimen.

When the six-month marker came around, all her symptoms had completely resolved, her thyroid levels were normal, and TPO antibodies remained under 100, which showed Hashimoto's was clinically in remission.

of 40 percent of the population are living with some level of underactive thyroid, known medically as hypothyroidism. The most common cause is Hashimoto's disease. Symptoms include chronic fatigue, weight gain, and low metabolism.

The majority of cases I've seen have been linked to some sort of dietary trigger, which is why all my Hashimoto's patients are tested for food immune reactions and leaky gut. The most common cross-reactive foods in this category are lectins and agglutinins, chief among them a wheat peptide called wheat germ agglutinin, or WGA. When I prescribe a gluten-free diet to my patients, most experience complete resolution. No studies have proven this scientifically, but when removing gluten from the diet, I've witnessed a reduction in TSH levels and normalized thyroid antibodies. This often leads to lowering or completely eliminating the need for medication.

On the other end of the thyroid spectrum is hyperthyroidism, and Graves' disease is the most common form. Two rare cases involve President George H.W. Bush and his wife Barbara. Barbara was diagnosed with Graves' in 1989, followed by George in 1991. "Conjugal Graves' disease" is the medical term to describe partners who are both diagnosed with this hyperthyroid immune disorder. Rather than mere coincidence, as one physician at Walter Reed Hospital had suggested, it appears more likely that the presidential couple came into contact with a virus, too much iodine in their diet, or some sort of environmental toxin. Curiously enough, a third member of their family—their pet English springer spaniel Millie—was diagnosed with lupus.

Graves' is not as dire as it sounds. Named after the nineteenth-century surgeon Robert J. Graves, who discovered the condition, it is one of the easiest hormone disorders to cure when armed with the right information.

COMMON AUTOIMMUNE THYROIDITIS CONDITIONS

Which form of autoimmune thyroiditis develops depends on the autoantibody your immune system produces. If it binds to the receptors on the thyroid gland, then Graves' will follow. If the autoantibodies target enzymes that slow production of thyroid hormone, Hashimoto's will ensue.

Graves' disease (a form of hyperthyroidism) is an autoimmune condition that causes your thyroid to

KNOW THE SIGNS

When autoimmunity attacks the thyroid, you may experience:

Graves' disease (a form of hyperthyroidism)

- Anxiety
- Difficulty sleeping
- Frequent bowel movements
- Heat sensitivity
- Hyperactivity
- Irregular heartbeat
- Protruding eyes
- Rapid heart rate
- Sweating
- Tremors
- Weight loss

Hashimoto's thyroiditis (a form of hypothyroidism)

- Aches and pains
- Constipation
- Depression
- Dry skin and brittle nails
- Extreme fatigue
- Forgetfulness
- Hair loss
- Intolerance to cold
- Weight gain

Risk Factors

- Certain medications (amiodarone and interferon)
- Environmental toxins
- Genetic predisposition
- High levels of iodine (Graves')
- Infections (human herpesvirus 6/HHV-6, Epstein-Barr virus/EBV, SARS-CoV2/COVID-19, yersiniosis)
- Radiation
- Smoking
- Stress

Common Trigger Foods in This Category

- Beans
- Corn
- Dairy
- Eggs
- Wheat
- Soy
- Spinach
- Tomato

produce too much T4 hormone and affects about 1 percent of Americans. Graves' develops when autoantibodies called thyroid-stimulating immunoglobulins (TSI) land on receptors in the thyroid gland and tell the thyroid to keep producing more. As a result, the thyroid floods the bloodstream with T4 without any input from the pituitary gland. The immune response causes inflammation and abnormal deposits in the muscles, including the connecting muscles behind the eyes. Drugs like methimazole are prescribed to suppress the thyroid. When drugs don't work, the thyroid is often surgically removed or treated with radioactive iodine. Symptoms include hair loss, weight loss, anxiety, palpitations, rapid heart rate, and diarrhea. About 30 percent of all cases may develop exophthalmos, or bulging eye, a condition that causes the eyes to push forward from their sockets.

Hashimoto's thyroiditis, the most common form of an underactive thyroid and the main cause of hypothyroidism, develops when the thyroid does not make enough T4. This is caused by autoantibodies binding to thyroid peroxidase (TPO), an essential enzyme in the thyroid responsible for making T4 and T3. Symptoms include sensitivity to cold, chronic fatigue, memory problems, achiness, depression, dry skin, hair loss, and weight gain. To replace the hormone the thyroid is no longer producing, synthetic hormones like levothyroxine are often prescribed under the brand names Synthroid and Levoxyl. Hashimoto's can cause various organs in the body to break down, inducing other autoimmune diseases such as rheumatoid arthritis and lupus.

Recommended Tests

- Array 2: Intestinal Antigenic Permeability Screen (Cyrex Laboratories)
- Array 3X: Wheat/Gluten Proteome Reactivity and Autoimmunity (Cyrex Laboratories)
- Array 4: Gluten-Associated Cross-Reactive Foods and Foods Sensitivity (Cyrex Laboratories)
- Thyroid Peroxidase and Thyroglobulin Test (Labcorp or Quest Diagnostics)
- TSHRab or Thyroid Stimulating Immunoglobulin (Labcorp or Quest Diagnostics)

With these tests, we're looking for high serum levels of autoantibodies against thyroid peroxidase (TPO), an enzyme that plays a critical role in the production of T4 and T3. It's worth noting that not everyone with Hashimoto's tests positive for TPO and many others who don't have Hashimoto's show TPO. Still, it's a good place to start. We also look for thyroglobulin (TG), which is commonly detected in autoimmune thyroiditis. A third autoantibody, the TSH receptor antibody (TSHRab), also known as thyroid-stimulating immunoglobulin, is detected in Graves' disease but is negative in Hashimoto's.

8

THE JOINTS

We've all got stardust in our bones.

– Ben Harper, singer-songwriter

The body contains 206 bones, and wherever they meet, you'll find a joint. Joints outnumber bones—on average, everyone has about 360—but not all are similar. The immovable joints that sit between the plates of the skull, for example, are called synarthroses. Amphiarthroses joints are found between the bones of the spine and move slightly, like for bending over or doing backbends.

Most joints, however, are the movable synovial joints, found in the hands, feet, shoulders, hips, knees, and elbows. These marvelous works of engineering cushion bones with smooth cartilage and are lubricated by an egg white–like substance called synovial fluid. This allows you to move with ease in a variety of ways, from getting up out of a chair to performing a tango. When your immune system goes haywire and strikes these areas, however, you end up with stiff, achy, and swollen joints that slow you down and disrupt daily life. Severe cases can mean joint erosion and internal organ damage.

The Arthritis Foundation estimates that 92.1 million adults in the U.S. have either arthritic symptoms or doctor-diagnosed arthritis. Arthritis—"arth" for joints and "itis" for inflammation—is an umbrella term covering more than 100 types of a musculoskeletal illnesses. For our purposes, however, we'll focus on the types caused by autoimmunity.

Rheumatoid arthritis (RA)—the most common form of autoimmune arthritis, affecting 1.5 million adults in the U.S.—is frequently found in patients with irritable bowel disorder (IBD). What's more, those living with celiac disease are often found to have rheumatoid arthritis or a form of psoriasis that resides in the joints called psoriatic arthritis

In 2017, the Brigham RA Sequential Study (BRASS), reported that nearly one-quarter of its 217 subjects with longstanding RA found significant improvement after changing their diets. Foods such as blueberries and spinach decreased symptoms, while sugary sodas and desserts worsened them. It's no surprise that refined sugar escalated symptoms, as it's one of the most inflammatory foods on the planet. When you

CASE STUDY: RICHARD

Richard, a fifty-nine-year-old man, had been experiencing migratory arthritis, affecting his shoulders first, then moving to his elbows, left hip, and right knee. He also reported chronic diarrhea for two and a half years with a colonoscopy that came back negative and a standard lab report for rheumatoid arthritis that was also negative. Richard's rheumatologist told him they did not know the cause of his arthritis. That's when he arrived at my clinic.

Detect the problem: I tested Richard for nutritional deficiencies and autoimmunity of the joints. I also wanted to rule out leaky gut and food reactivity, since leaky gut is the gateway to autoimmune disorders, and Richard was clearly dealing with one. Because foods represent the most common trigger for leaky gut, I tested him for gluten, wheat germ agglutinin, dairy, and egg reactivity, and he tested positive for all of them.

Remove the triggers: Based on Richard's test results, we eliminated gluten, dairy, and egg from his diet.

Repair the barrier: I put Richard on probiotics to help heal the gut barrier, turmeric to reduce inflammation, and fish oil to relieve his tender joints and ease morning stiffness. Because he had low vitamin D levels, we also added vitamin D (5,000 IU daily). Vitamin D is not actually a vitamin but a hormone and is particularly beneficial in cases like Richard's, as it helps balance immune function and diminish autoimmunity.

Results: Within three months, Richard was asymptomatic and successfully avoided the use of biologics and joint replacement surgery. His bowel habits also became more regular, and he reported improved energy and mental clarity. By eliminating Richard's triggers, his inflammation ceased.

overindulge, your immune system mistakenly sends T cells to your joints, where they release pro-inflammatory cytokines. In inflammatory arthritis, cytokine levels are already high, so adding sugar is throwing fuel on a fire. Eating sugar can further alter the gut microbiome, allowing the release of lipopolysaccharides into the bloodstream, where it can enter joint spaces and increase inflammation and pain.

Even seemingly healthy foods like beans, lentils, tomatoes, peppers, and eggplant can be problematic for people with arthritis. These and other foods contain lectins, which can lead to an onset of rheumatoid arthritis. When lectins (covered more in Chapter 13), are not properly digested and their molecules escape into the bloodstream, they latch on to red blood cells. Once there, the lectin proteins are ushered throughout the body, leaving a wake of harm in their path. We see the most damage in collagen and joint connective tissue.

Lectins are also known to bind to the CD161 receptor on natural killer cells (NK) and appear to have a role in driving inflammation in the joints. Finally, lectins can bind to major components of the joints known as glycosaminoglycans and proteoglycans. In fact, lectin injected into mice was found to bind to immunoglobulin G antibodies and cause RA.

Other dietary culprits are gluten and dairy. Their proteins can cross-react with joint tissue and cause alterations in a process known as citrullination. Basically, citrullination occurs when the amino acid arginine is converted to another non-essential amino acid called citrulline. For people with RA, this process alters type-2 collagen.

Citrulline gets carried to the lymph nodes, where T-helper cells stimulate the B-cells to produce autoantibodies against the citrulline. Next, the T-helper cells and autoantibodies enter the bloodstream and head to the joints. In the joints, the T cells release inflammatory cytokines and recruit even more inflammatory cells called macrophages to the site. (Macrophages are like the Pac-Man of the immune system that gobble up harmful organisms. They also produce inflammatory cytokines.) So now the joint area is receiving inflammatory responses from several sources—T cells, autoantibodies, and macrophages—and it's a perfect storm.

As a result, the synovial cells in your joints try to ward off the attack by proliferating, and the increased synovial and immune cells create a thick, swollen synovial membrane. Over time, cartilage wears away and bones begin to erode and rub against each other. This is why it is so important to test for citrullinated peptides if you are dealing with RA.

Traditional medical advice remains focused on masking RA pain with steroids, painkilling medications, and sometimes surgery. Unfortunately, these treatments do not address or remove the root cause of the inflammation, nor do they restore joint function.

If you are living with autoimmune arthritis, be aware that pectin-rich fruit such as cooking apples, crab apples, black currants, cranberries, gooseberries, plums, oranges, lemons, and quince may play a role in the development of joint disorders. Use them sparingly and take note if they aggravate your symptoms. Additionally, glycine-rich foods like gelatin, meat, soy protein, chicken, eggs, seeds, cereals, French beans, and rice may also cross-react with collagen and keratin. Undercooked pork is also problematic, as it can transmit *Yersinia enterocolitica* bacteria and cause reactive arthritis and joint issues, so I generally tell my patients with these conditions (including rheumatoid arthritis and Guillain-Barré syndrome) to avoid pork altogether. If you choose to eat pork, make sure to select pasture-raised and without nitrates.

Consider adding a wide variety of organic vegetables and low-glycemic fruits to your diet. They contain natural anti-inflammatory compounds and are rich sources of fiber. Cold-water fatty fish are also beneficial. The omega-3 fatty acids in salmon, trout, mackerel, and herring help reduce inflammation and ease morning stiffness. You can also try fish oil supplements, but always talk to your doctor first, as higher doses can interact with some drugs, including medications for high blood pressure.

Finally, regular exercise such as walking, water aerobics, and low-impact aerobics are especially beneficial for range of motion in the joints.

TYPES OF INFLAMMATORY ARTHRITIS

Inflammatory arthritis is typically triggered by a genetic factor set off by something in the environment. For instance, a person with a gene for human leukocyte antigen (HLA-DL1 and HLA-DL4) might develop rheumatoid arthritis after exposure to a toxin like cigarette smoke or a specific intestinal pathogen like *salmonella, Shigella,* and *Yersinia.* The appearance of immunoglobulin M antibodies against *Proteus mirabilis,* a species of bacteria found in the urinary tract, also

NOTES FROM THE LAB

With autoimmunity, the immune system is always running on high speed, flooding the body with cytokine inflammatory signals that ultimately result in joint and tissue damage. Standard treatment for autoimmune joint diseases such as rheumatoid arthritis, psoriatic arthritis, and ankylosing spondylitis include immunosuppressants like Plaquenil or methotrexate, as well as a class of medications known as biologics. Collectively these medications are referred to as disease-modifying antirheumatic drugs, or DMARDs.

Biologics work by binding to cytokines and removing them from the bloodstream, along with the symptoms. While that sounds great, biologics are basically synthetic antibodies designed to block chemical signals that have a real purpose, and they remove a functional arm of the immune system. As a result, patients become prone to infection and are at higher risk for developing leukemia, lymphoma, and melanoma. In my practice, I like to consider all treatment options available—DMARDs, lifestyle intervention, and supplements. My goal is always to minimize or possibly eliminate the need for medication as part of a treatment protocol, though sometimes they remain helpful and essential.

KNOW THE SIGNS

When autoimmunity attacks the joints, you may experience:

- Fatigue and weakness
- Fluid in the joints
- Joint pain
- Lack of appetite
- Loss of mobility in the joints
- Low-grade fever
- Nodules that grow beneath the skin near the joint
- Stiffness (usually worse in the mornings)
- Swelling

Risk Factors

- Bacterial or viral infections
- Environmental toxins such as smoke, insecticides, and air pollution
- Exposure to cigarette smoke early in life
- Gender
- Genetics
- Obesity
- Poor diet
- Smoking
- Stress

Common Trigger Foods in This Category

- Dairy
- Gluten
- Grains
- Lectins
- Sugar
- Pork

Recommended Tests

- Test for rheumatoid factor and citrullinated peptides (Labcorp and Quest Diagnostics)
- Array 2: Intestinal Antigenic Permeability Screen 3 (Cyrex Laboratories)
- Array 8: Joint Autoimmune Reactivity Screen (Cyrex Laboratories)
- Array 10: Multiple Food Immune Reactivity Screen (Cyrex Laboratories)

Surprisingly, rheumatoid factor (RF)—recognized as the classic autoantibody for rheumatoid arthritis for more than seventy years—is not actually the ideal diagnostic biomarker for the disease. While rheumatoid factors are often detected in the elderly, in other autoimmune diseases, and with certain infectious diseases, the number is relatively low in rheumatoid arthritis patients.

suggests a pathogenic relationship to rheumatoid arthritis. Likewise, antibodies against the oral bacteria *P. gingivalis*, found in dental infections, have also been linked to the onset of rheumatoid arthritis because they cause citrullination of proteins.

Autoimmune arthritis includes a number of subtypes, including rheumatoid arthritis, systemic lupus erythematosus (SLE or lupus), Sjögren's syndrome, and psoriatic arthritis. Many forms commonly involve multiple body systems, including the skin, lungs, eyes, heart, and blood vessels. Here are some of the most common arthritis subtypes that fall under the autoimmune umbrella.

Juvenile idiopathic arthritis affects an estimated 300,000 children in the United States. Symptoms include joint pain, eye inflammation, fevers, and rashes. According to the National Institute of Arthritis and Musculoskeletal and Skin Diseases, patients with juvenile idiopathic arthritis experience increased intestinal permeability along with gastrointestinal symptoms, suggesting a role for intestinal changes in the pathogenesis of rheumatic diseases.

Psoriatic arthritis (PsA) affects an estimated 8 million Americans and causes skin cells to multiply at a much quicker rate, producing itchy, scaly rashes and patches of dry skin—typically on the scalp, elbows, knees, and lower back, but they can be found almost anywhere on the body, including fingers and toes. It also causes weak nails. About 30 percent of patients with psoriasis also develop PsA. The presence of psoriasis, inflammatory arthritis, and absence of positive serological tests for rheumatoid arthritis are the hallmarks of PsA. The disease can lay dormant in the body until triggered by an outside influence such as infection. Conventional treatment typically involves topical or oral medication designed only to mask the inflammation.

Rheumatoid arthritis (RA) is the most common form of inflammatory arthritis, and it affects upwards of 1.5 million Americans, with women three times more likely to get it than men. RA can begin between the ages of thirty and fifty, but it may take years for the debilitating symptoms to take hold. It is usually seen on both sides of the body and affects the joints of the hands, feet, wrists, elbows, knees, and ankles. If left unchecked, RA can progress from swollen, achy joints to damaged cartilage, erosion of the nearby bones, and shrinkage in the joint space. Anti-inflammatory medications are typically prescribed, but they don't always work for everyone. The Arthritis Foundation reports that in 2015, the national indirect costs of RA-related absenteeism from work were $252 million.

Sjögren's syndrome affects the exocrine glands that produce moisture in the body, causing dryness of the eyes, mouth, and other body parts. The disease can also cause inflammatory arthritis, abnormally dry skin, Raynaud's disease, nerve damage, and disorders of the esophagus, stomach, intestines, liver, and pancreas, as well as voice-related disorders. The condition can also appear alongside thyroid disease and rheumatoid arthritis, and in 20 percent of cases, patients experience neurological issues. Four million Americans are estimated to be living with the condition.

Spondyloarthritis (SpA) is an umbrella term for autoimmune disorders that affect the joints, tendons, and ligaments. The most common in this category is ankylosing spondylitis, a type of arthritis that causes pain and stiffness in the spinal joints. This form tends to affect men more often than women and is responsible for up to 5 percent of all patients complaining of back pain. Comorbidities in this category include psoriatic arthritis; reactive arthritis, which presents with joint pain, red eyes, burning with urination, or a rash on the palms of the hands or soles of the feet and commonly occurs in those who have a history of certain bacterial infections such as *chlamydia, salmonella, Shigella,* or *campylobacter*; and enteropathic arthritis, which is associated with inflammatory bowel disease.

With SpA, joint inflammation often comes and goes and is accompanied by fatigue. Other symptoms include osteoporosis, pain and redness of the eye, inflammation of the aortic heart valve, and intestinal inflammation. Typical treatments include NSAIDs and physical therapy.

Systemic lupus erythematosus (SLE) accounts for about 70 percent of all lupus cases and affects the entire body, including the joints, kidneys, skin, blood, brain, and other organs. Symptoms include fever, rash, fatigue, depression, joint pain, brain fog, hair loss, headaches, anemia, stomach and bowel issues, sensitivity to light, increased susceptibility to infections, blood-clotting problems, and more. In the United States, more than 1.5 million people are living with SLE. Women between the ages of fifteen and forty-four are at the greatest risk of developing the disease, though up to 20 percent of new cases develop before age eighteen.

Since SLE affects the entire body with many symptoms, diagnosis is often difficult. Because there is no genetic component with SLE, it's even trickier. One telltale sign, however, is a prominent red "butterfly rash" that appears on the face. Researchers believe that diet, stress, trauma, viruses, certain medications, and ultraviolet rays may trigger its onset. Conventional treatment typically involves anti-inflammatory drugs such as corticosteroids, steroid creams, and hydroxychloroquine.

9

THE SKIN

Beauty is being comfortable and confident in your own skin.

– Iman Abdulmajid, fashion model

The skin is a window to the immune system, reflecting on the outside what's going on within. If your gut is healthy, it reveals itself on your skin, clear and glowing, without blemishes and neither flaky nor dry. But if there's inflammation in your intestinal lining, you may experience inflammation on your skin as well.

Like your gut, your skin is charged with preventing foreign substances from entering your body. And like your gut, your skin is home to a unique microbiome teeming with trillions of bacteria. Just like the beneficial bugs in your gut, the good microbes on your skin play a critical role in maintaining balance by inhibiting the growth of invading pathogens. It also informs your immune system whenever you come in contact with new microbes.

The association between the gut and skin is so strong, there's even a term for it: the gut-skin axis, akin to the gut-brain axis. The cells lining your intestinal tract are very similar to skin cells, and these cells are in constant communication with each other, mostly by way of the immune system to help regulate inflammation. Expectant mothers experience a "pregnancy glow," and many women go through the occasional breakout during their menstrual periods and in the years leading up to menopause. These are all examples of the gut communicating the body's hormonal levels. Perhaps you've heard of people whose skin took on an orange hue after drinking too much carrot juice. This, too, demonstrates how the gut communicates nutrients to the skin—in this case, an excess of beta-carotene.

Ample evidence shows autoimmune diseases of the skin frequently show up alongside other autoimmune conditions. Some are related to the overproduction of cytokines, while others are linked to molecular mimicry.

In recent years, researchers have become increasingly interested in the gut-skin connection. In fact, some physicians are treating psoriasis with the same treatment used to treat Crohn's, with an immunosuppressive drug called ustekinumab (brand name Stelara). Emerging evidence also links small intestinal bacterial

---

CASE STUDY: LORI

Lori, a twenty-nine-year-old woman, came to me with a lifelong history of eczema behind the ears, along the shins, and in the creases of her elbows and knees. She had had persistent asthma since age eight and developed skin conditions later in life. Multiple doctors treated the eczema with topical steroids, but she began seeing an acupuncturist for Chinese herbs when nothing cured her. The Eastern approach resulted in improvement for a couple of months, but Lori's skin problems eventually returned. She also reported mild abdominal pain and daily multiple loose bowel movements containing undigested food particles.

Detect the problem: Lori clearly had issues with her digestive tract, so we tested for leaky gut, which came back positive. Further tests revealed non-celiac gluten sensitivity, gut dysbiosis, and an intolerance to dairy.

Remove the triggers: Lori eliminated gluten and dairy from her diet.

Repair the barrier: We added a 100 billion CFU lacto-bifido probiotic, 2.3 grams fish oil once a day, 5,000 IU vitamin D, short chain fatty acids (EnteroVite by Apex Energetics), and RepairVite (by Apex Energetics), along with therapeutic topical zinc and oatmeal ointment.

Results: After three months, Lori reported that her eczema had completely healed. What's more, her bowel movements normalized and her asthma had gone into remission.

---

overgrowth (SIBO) with rosacea. People with SIBO are ten times more likely to have a skin issue, and disorders are also prevalent in those with celiac disease. Dermatitis herpetiformis, an autoimmune skin disease, for instance, is caused by a reaction to gluten, so it's no coincidence that it is often seen alongside celiac.

Food glue made from transglutaminase is another problem. In this form, the enzyme is used as an additive and acts as a protein glue in meat and baked goods (particularly gluten-free products). Its purpose is to extend shelf life and glue smaller pieces of meat together. Though the amino acid sequences between tissue transglutaminase and "food glue" transglutaminase are not exact, they are close enough that molecular mimicry can and does ensue, particularly among those with gut and skin issues. (We'll discuss transglutaminase as a food additive in more detail in Chapter 14.)

Repairing the skin has more to do with healing your interior environment than applying topical treatments. It starts with removing specific dietary triggers and restoring the gut with supplements such as vitamin D and high-potency probiotics containing *lactobacilli* and *Bifidobacterium*. Fish oil is good, too, since it acts as an intestinal anti-inflammatory and helps with skin integrity. And finally, I like glutathione, taken intermittently, three months on and one month off. When taken orally, glutathione helps relax inflammation in the gut, where it all starts.

INFLAMMATORY AND AUTOIMMUNE SKIN CONDITIONS

While our ancient ancestors understood that the appearance of our skin is a reflection of the deeper workings of our body, they were not exposed to processed food, pollution, and genetically modified organisms. These modern hazards wreak havoc on the body's natural balance, which then manifest through various skin disorders. Listed here are some of the more common autoimmune skin disorders.

Eczema affects more than 30 million Americans. The word "eczema" has Greek origins and means "to boil over." It's a harsh metaphor, but that is essentially what is taking place: inflammation boils over into the epidermal layers and protrudes onto the outer layers, presenting itself as dry, itchy, patchy skin. With eczema, immunoglobulin A (IgA)- or immunoglobulin M (IgM)-mediated food immune reactivity are at play. Many people with eczema also experience food sensitivities and intolerances from a GI response that evolves into the skin disorder. IgA antibodies break through the intestinal lining and bind to the epidermal transglutaminase (tTG-3), causing localized inflammation. With egg and milk allergies, histamines are produced as an immunoglobulin E (IgE)-mediated response that can lead to skin reactions such as eczema or acne.

Dermatitis herpetiformis (DH) is an autoimmune disorder in which IgA antibodies made against gluten and epidermal transglutaminase 3 (tTG-3) attack enzymes in the skin. Often misdiagnosed as eczema, the condition causes clusters of extremely itchy blisters and raised red lesions that resemble acne. It shows up asymmetrically on the elbows, knees, buttocks, lower back, and scalp. Genetics and gluten sensitivity play significant roles in onset of DH, and it is often found in people who have celiac disease. Traditional treatment consists of a strict gluten-free diet and anti-inflammatory medications like Dapsone.

Discoid lupus erythematosus (DLE) manifests as crusty, purple-red disc-shaped lesions on the cheeks, nose, ears, scalp, and hands but can sometimes show up in other areas of the body. Lesions often lose skin pigment and can be itchy or tender. DLE appears to have a genetic factor and is five times more common in women than men. It also tends to be more severe in smokers than nonsmokers. Traditional treatments include cortisone ointment and injections, hydroxychloroquine, Accutane, or Soriatane.

Hidradenitis suppurativa attacks the apocrine glands (a type of sweat gland) and is characterized by inflamed clusters of lesions and painful, pus-filled boils, typically in areas that have skin-to-skin contact such as under the armpits, under the breasts, the groin area, and inner thighs. Treatments typically involve NSAIDs and oral and topical antibiotics. The condition is more common in women and African Americans.

Idiopathic urticaria is a fancy term for hives. Allergies to nuts, chocolate, seafood, tomatoes, eggs, fresh berries, dairy, insect stings, and certain medications can cause urticaria. The condition is typically related to IgE-mediated allergies and caused by a release of histamine and other proinflammatory mediators. But 30 to 40 percent of chronic idiopathic urticaria is autoimmune and is often associated with autoimmune thyroid disease.

Lichen planus is characterized by shiny, reddish-purple, flat-topped bumps that often have an angular shape. The disease can occur anywhere on the skin, but often favors the inside of the wrists and ankles, the lower legs, back, and neck. In some people, the mouth, genital region, hair, and nails are affected. Thick patches may occur, especially on the shins, and, though rare, the condition can also produce blisters. Bumps may appear in areas of trauma on some people. About 20 percent of the time, lichen planus of the skin causes minimal symptoms and needs no treatment. However, in many cases, the itching can be constant and intense. This disease occurs most often in men and women between the ages of thirty and seventy.

Psoriasis results when T cells mistakenly attack skin cells. This causes skin cells to grow up to ten times faster than normal, causing a buildup of red, itchy, scaly patches on the scalp, elbows, knees and lower back. In the U.S., about 7.4 million people are living with the condition. Ten percent of the population inherit the gene that can lead to psoriasis; however, only 2 percent go on to develop it. Food is a prevailing trigger that turns on the gene. Conventional treatment typically involves topical or oral medication designed only to mask the inflammation.

Scleroderma is a group of inflammatory connective tissue disorders that cause a thickening of the skin (a process known as fibrosis). Internal organs and blood vessels can also become damaged. The condition usually starts with a few dry patches on the hands or face that gradually become thicker and spread to other areas of the body.

KNOW THE SIGNS

When autoimmunity attacks the skin, you may experience:

- Hives
- Itching
- Rashes
- Redness
- Scaling
- Swelling

Common Trigger Foods in This Category

- Corn
- Dairy
- Eggs
- Wheat and gluten-containing grains
- Carrot, soybean, and spinach (for lupus)

Risk Factors

- Birth via C-section
- Early/frequent antibiotic use
- History of seasonal allergies or asthma
- Poor diet during childhood

Recommended Tests

- Array 2: Intestinal Antigenic Permeability Screen (Cyrex Laboratories)
- Array 3X: Wheat/Gluten Proteome Reactivity and Autoimmunity (Cyrex Laboratories)

The vast majority of skin-related autoimmune disorders are linked to gluten reactivity and leaky gut, so I found these two arrays are the best place to start. On Array 3, I'm looking specifically for a unique marker called transglutaminase-3 (tTG3). For cases where lupus is suspected, I look for antibodies that react with ribonucleoprotein particles, which cross-react with common food proteins such as soybean, corn, spinach, and carrot. By removing these foods, the disease course of lupus can be improved. The blood serum of many patients with scleroderma cross-reacts with plant enzymes found in wheat germ, peas, corn, and spinach.

Vitiligo occurs when T cells attack melanocytes, the cells that produce melanin and provide color to the skin. This results in patches of skin—and sometimes hair—losing pigmentation. More than 2 million Americans are living with the condition, and up to 30 percent of women with vitiligo develop autoimmune thyroid disorders. Other autoimmune comorbidities include alopecia areata, Addison's disease, pernicious anemia, and diabetes mellitus.

PART III:
REMOVE THE TRIGGERS

10

SMOOTHING THE TRANSITION

Your positive action combined with positive thinking results in success.

– Shive Khera, author

During the food elimination phase, most people notice improvements within the first two weeks. Even so, it often takes up to six weeks to feel a significant change. This is because the autoantibodies to your trigger foods have a half-life of up to three weeks, meaning that you'll continue to experience some level of inflammation for a while. Peak improvements from dietary removals typically occur at about three months, so please be patient with your progress. I can't tell you how many times a patient of mine wanted to quit at the one-month mark. Once they had a bit more time under their belts, though, they found a new respect for fueling their bodies with the right types of food.

I also want to stress that certain foods are highly addictive, causing you to go through withdrawal. After removing sugar, for instance, you may experience headaches and moodiness. Similarly, gluten and dairy contain opiate peptides that can cause similar (yet not as severe) effects to an opiate withdrawal. You may feel a temporary decrease in energy or even an increase in overall pain that typically passes in about a week. As you eliminate the toxins in your body, you may also experience other minor symptoms such as constipation, light-headedness, moodiness, or a pimple or two. The good news is withdrawal symptoms pass around the third week, and on the other side awaits brilliant health.

If you're overweight, you may lose some pounds. If you're severely underweight, you may gain. You might notice boundless energy and feel like taking on a big project, an ambitious new job, or decide to go back to school and earn another degree. You may feel so great, in fact, that you'll be tempted to backslide and sample one of your beloved trigger foods. Beware: Your body will resist, often with a flare-up too loud to ignore. You might even feel like these former favorite foods are poison. For you, they are. If you end up backsliding, simply get back on the program. After a few weeks, the foods you once desired will begin to lose their allure, and you might not even miss them at all once your body is back in balance.

PRACTICAL TIPS

When you remove trigger foods from your diet, you are essentially resetting your body from inflammation and oxidative stress, which occurs when free radicals outnumber antioxidants. The key here is to be patient with yourself, monitor your symptoms, and by all means, dive into activities that point you closer to your health goals. Here are a few action items to get started.

Plan your meals in advance. Precut organic veggies for salads, stir-fries, and soups, and place quick snacks like celery sticks and baby carrots front and center in your fridge. For smoothies, cut and freeze your ingredients in advance and store them in a tempered glass container made specially for freezing. Speaking of the freezer, fill it with bags of organic cauliflower, broccoli, and kale. Roast veggies like sweet potatoes, brussels sprouts, or kale chips in advance so they're handy throughout the week. Batch cook meals with lean proteins such as wild-caught salmon, halibut, trout, grass-fed burgers, or pasture-raised chicken. Don't forget about homemade soups and bone broth—you can freeze the leftovers for later. Be sure to have sprouts on hand for topping your salads and romaine lettuce for a bread or tortilla substitute. For a sweet bite, keep pints of low-glycemic fruits like strawberries, blueberries, or cherries on hand.

Stay hydrated. Your body requires proper hydration to transport nutrients to your cells and organs. Be sure to drink plenty of filtered water. Other healing options include herbal teas, tonics, and bone broths. You can make your water more interesting by adding lemon or cucumber slices, or even a sprig of rosemary. Fruit juices contain too much sugar, so I do not recommend those. Celery juice, however, is highly beneficial and is known to reduce inflammation.

Hit the farmers market. Get to know the good people who grow and raise your food. The produce at farmers markets tends to be local and in season, and fresher and less expensive than what you might find at your local supermarket. Depending on your city, many farmers also sell wild-caught fish and grass-fed meats.

Up your exercise. If you're feeling an energy drain shortly after eliminating your trigger foods, you may want to take it easy. It's OK to rest, but continue to move your body. Head out for a walk, dance in your living room, or take an online yoga or tai chi class. If you feel up to it, lift some weights or do some cardio. Studies show that exercise increases the transport of oxygen through the body, including the gut, which in turn promotes healthy microbes. Another study shows that a chemical called brain-derived neurotrophic factor (BDNF) increases in the body during exercise.

BDNF tells neurons to grow and correlates with improvements in cognitive functions. It also reduces your risk of cardiovascular disease and Alzheimer's. Yet another study has shown that exercise increases the number of stem cells in the bone marrow. Stem cells have the potential to become other types of cells, including T and B cells. For this reason, they are known as the mother of all other cells and serve a biological repair function in a healthy immune system.

Connect with nature. You may find yourself thinking about food more than usual during this time. I can think of no better diversion than leaving your cell phone behind and heading outdoors to soak up some fresh air and sunshine, or gazing at the stars at night. If the weather's less than ideal, put on a raincoat and head outside anyway. This is a great opportunity to slow down, observe, and pay attention to nuances you might have overlooked before. This is particularly important for city dwellers. A 2014 study in Japan shows that when we immerse ourselves in natural surroundings, like a forest, we lower our stress levels and enhance the function of our natural killer cells.

Laughter is the best medicine. Watch a comedy, tune into a funny cat video on YouTube, or amuse your friends and family by making silly faces and impersonations. Studies find that a good hearty laugh strengthens the immune system, improves mood, releases feel-good hormones like endorphins, and reduces pain, stress, and inflammation.

Meditate toward better health. Stress is one of the five major factors contributing to autoimmune disorders. In an eight-week study developed in the 1970s by the Stress Reduction Clinic at UMass Medical Center, researchers discovered that meditation promotes emotional health, improves sleep, and provides relief from stress, pain, depression, and illness.

Listen to music. A wealth of studies over the last decade has shown that listening to music can enhance immune function, boost energy, improve mood and memory, regulate emotions, reduce stress, ease pain, decrease depression, and produce a sense of calm.

Give yourself a dry brush massage. A type of Ayurvedic medicine, dry brush massage promotes blood circulation, enhances immune function, and promotes lymph flow by excreting toxins and invigorating the nervous system. It also helps open the pores and exfoliate the skin. The best time to perform a dry brush massage is in the morning, before your shower. Start at the toes and brush in long strokes toward your heart. The process should take two or three minutes. Be sure to purchase a brush with coarse, natural-fiber bristles instead of synthetic ones, as the latter can be harsh on the skin. If you have a skin condition, please exercise caution and avoid affected areas.

Pamper yourself. Head to the spa or create a spa environment at home. Enjoy a massage, get a pedicure, or luxuriate in a steam room or your steamy bathroom. The idea here is to experience pure indulgence without guilt.

Prioritize sleep. Poor sleep can bring on cravings for carbs, make you cranky, and affect your memory. Over the long term, chronic lack of sleep is associated with weight gain, diabetes, hypertension, heart attack, and stroke. Be sure to get between seven and nine hours of uninterrupted sleep each night.

Take an Epsom salt bath. Loaded with magnesium, Epsom salt baths relax the mind, soothe achy muscles, soften skin, and relieve stress, anxiety, and depression. A 2010 study also found that soaking in a tub with Epsom

NOTES FROM THE LAB

If you've learned about your triggers before serious symptoms set in, congratulate yourself! With the power of science, observation, and common sense, you've redirected your path toward glowing health. Even if you are currently living with the effects of a full-blown, active autoimmune disease, you'll notice dramatic improvements and an enhanced quality of life once you remove the foods causing inflammation in your body.

salt increases your serotonin levels. Epsom salt baths may even help you sleep better. Make yours extra special by adding a few drops of lavender essential oil.

Foster healthy relationships. The company we keep is just as important as the foods we eat. Both can have profound effects on our health and mental well-being. Surround yourself with supportive people who have similar goals, enjoy eating clean foods, and participate in healthy pursuits.

Detox and declutter. As you clean your body from the inside, reflect those positive, healing changes in your external surroundings as well. A tidy environment lessens allergies, reduces anxiety, enhances confidence, and energizes the spirit. Toss out the old magazines, eliminate plastics in your kitchen wherever possible, comb through your clothes and donate what you no longer wear. Remove toxic products containing phthalates, perchloroethylene, and triclosan, too—this includes dryer sheets and perfumed soaps and air fresheners. Think of decluttering as opening your mind to new possibilities.

Read motivational books. Research shows that reading reduces stress, strengthens brain connections, enhances compassion, and improves vocabulary. If you struggle with falling asleep, try turning off the TV, powering down your electronic devices, and curling up with a good book an hour before bedtime, especially those designed to empower your mind, body, and spirit. I've listed some of my favorites in the Resource section at the back of this book.

Adopt an attitude of gratitude. It's a scientific fact: Gratitude improves your physical and mental health. According to a 2012 study, grateful people experience fewer aches and pains, reduced aggressions and toxic emotions, increased happiness, improved self-esteem, enhanced sensitivity, and generally feeling healthy. Studies have even found that gratitude helps relieve emotions associated with trauma.

11

GLUTEN AND GRAINS

*Everyone should try no gluten for a week! The change in your skin,
physical and mental health is amazing. You won't go back!*

– Miley Cyrus

Humans have been cultivating cereal grains since the ancient days of the Fertile Crescent. Composed of up to 15 percent plant protein and 75 percent starch, grains such as wheat, spelt, and barley have served as excellent sources of calories and energy throughout much of human civilization, roughly 10,000 years. During times of scarcity, grains filled our bellies and helped keep the weight on. But it is wheat, of all grains, that emerged as the major staple crop across the globe, with about 5 billion people depending on it daily to round out their diets. In fact, world production exceeds 600 million tons a year.

Up until the second half of the twentieth century, wheat and other grains served as viable sustenance with no issues. So, why are so many of us now experiencing negative reactions—weight gain, digestive issues, brain fog, and joint pain, to name a few—from eating grains, specifically grains containing gluten, the binding protein that gives bread its scrumptious elasticity?

Enter the 1950s and the steady onslaught of synthetic fertilizers and chemical pesticides, insecticides, herbicides, and fungicides, added by the commercial food industry to help grains grow faster, hardier, and look "strong and healthy." Ideally a pesticide must be lethal enough to kill pests but not enough to affect humans. Sadly, this is not the case. We are beginning to understand that the excessive use of these chemical compounds is responsible for the rise in food immune reactivity and autoimmune disease—so much so that some are calling wheat the new tobacco. Epidemiological data shows a steady rise in autoimmune disease throughout the Western world over the last few decades, with evidence overwhelmingly pointing to environmental factors such as chemicals, infections, and food components over genetic factors.

In 1974, Monsanto introduced Roundup as a herbicide to replace the banned insecticide dichlorodiphenyltrichloroethane, commonly known as DDT. Since then, Roundup, or glyphosate, along

FOODS CONTAINING GLUTEN

When we think of gluten, most of us think of wheat, but it's found in a range of other grains as well, including rye, barley, triticale, and some oats. It's also in wheat varieties such as durum, emmer, semolina, spelt, farina, farro, graham, and einkorn—as well as everything from soy sauce to soups. The following list shows foods that may contain gluten. Be sure to check product labels and ask servers at restaurants.

- Baked goods like bread, pastries, biscuits, cake, cookies, and crackers
- Barbecue sauce (wheat is often found in Worcestershire sauce)
- Beer (unless explicitly labeled gluten-free)
- Breading and coating mixes
- Breakfast foods (like pancakes, waffles, crêpes, and French toast)
- Brewer's yeast
- Brown rice syrup
- Cereals
- Crackers (including communion wafers)
- Couscous
- Cream-based soups (sometimes thickened with flour)
- Croutons
- Energy bars
- Flour tortillas
- French fries (often either dusted with a gluten substance to become crispier or have shared the same oil bath as fried chicken, which is usually coated with flour batter)
- Granola
- Lunch meats
- Malt beverages
- Marinades (some contain soy sauce)
- Meat substitutes (manufacturers often use gluten to bind the ingredients)
- Medications and supplements (gluten is sometimes added to bind the ingredients)
- Multigrain chips
- Noodles
- Pastas
- Potato chips (some seasonings contain gluten)
- Pre-seasoned meats
- Salad dressings and marinades
- Sauces and gravies (roux, used to thicken gravy, is made with flour)
- Scrambled eggs served at restaurants (some restaurants add pancake batter to the mix)
- Self-basting poultry
- Soy sauce (note: tamari and liquid aminos made without wheat are gluten-free)
- Starch or dextrin
- Tortilla chips that are not entirely corn-based

with its cousin products, have become the most widely used pesticides in the United States. They are quite literally everywhere now—in the air, soil, water, in our meat and poultry, and, of course, massively present in our crops. This pesticide is extremely toxic, labeled by the World Health Organization (WHO) as "probably carcinogenic in humans." With the trillions of dollars at stake for the commercial food industry, Monsanto and Bayer continue to market this chemical. As it turns out, grains are the crop most heavily affected.

If food—in this case wheat—has been contaminated or polluted with chemicals, it can change to such an extent that the immune system no longer recognizes it as "friendly." Each person tolerates food differently. One person's genetics might allow them to alter their ability to tolerate wheat, while another's will identify that same wheat as a dangerous pathogen. For that person, continuing to eat wheat will trigger an ever-worsening cycle of inflammation throughout the body that can result in myriad disorders. Possibilities include autoimmunity and food immune reactivity that can spark brain fog, depression, chronic pain, joint degeneration, skin disorders, poor nutrition, and more.

Hybridized grains are another concern. Granted, hybridization has helped meet the demands of feeding a rapidly growing global population, which rose from 3 billion people in the 1960s to nearly 8 billion today. It also helps supply more feed for stock animals. Still, we now have more than 2,500 different types of wheat, all hybridized or crossbred from three varieties in just the past seventy years. If you don't think there is a danger in that, read on.

Conventional crossbreeding combines genes from varieties of wheat plants to produce new genetic combinations with different traits. This enhances the wheat's protein content and increases the proportion of lysine and tryptophan. While this results in a tastier and better-looking wheat, our digestive systems don't always recognize the new wheat peptides, so we are unequipped to digest them properly.

In response, a whopping 20 percent of the American population is experiencing a breakdown in their immune systems. Instead of recognizing the hybrid wheat as food, their immune systems perceive these new proteins as enemies and induce a loss of oral tolerance to wheat. What's more, wheat protein closely resembles proteins in human tissue, particularly the cerebellar component of the brain, so when the immune system attacks newer hybridized forms of wheat, it often attacks the brain and nervous system.

"Gluten-free" products are everywhere now because of the uptick in the allergic or immune response to gluten-containing products. This doesn't actually mean the gluten is removed from wheat, though. It actually means we are substituting wheat and other gluten grains such as rye, barley, spelt, and some oats with other ingredients. Gluten-free pastas are made with rice, corn, or lentil flour. Cookies sometimes use almond flour instead of all-purpose.

In some instances, these products are highly processed and contain food glues like transglutaminase or gums like xanthan that thicken and replicate the texture of gluten. Just because something is labeled gluten-free doesn't mean it's necessarily good for you, as transglutaminase and gums can be just as harmful as gluten itself. My quick rule of thumb: Try to stay away from gluten-free products that have more than one gum in them and avoid transglutaminase if you can. We'll discuss both of these in more detail in Chapter 14.

The number of people living with gluten allergies or intolerance is growing rapidly, and knowing how current farming practices manipulate wheat, it's difficult to argue that it's still "healthy" to consume, even if you don't have an immune reaction to it.

WHAT GLUTEN SENSITIVITY DOES TO YOUR BODY

What is gluten, exactly? Simply put, it's a protein with a very large molecule composed of several other proteins. In the digestive system, gluten is broken down into smaller peptides that get absorbed into the body through the small intestine. Some of these proteins—namely gliadin and glutenin—contain multiple amino acid sequences that can bind to similarly structured molecules in your body tissue and cause cross-reactivity, an example of molecular mimicry.

By creating antibodies against these proteins, the body also mistakenly attacks organs that are structurally similar. In patients with celiac and non-celiac gluten sensitivity, impacted organs typically include the brain (brain fog and headaches), skin (eczema or psoriasis), thyroid and hormones (autoimmune thyroiditis), and heart (coronary artery disease). Gluten sensitivity can also

TOP 10 SYMPTOMS OF GLUTEN IMMUNE REACTIVITY

- Bloating or cramping after meals
- Brain fog
- Chronic abdominal pain
- Chronic headaches
- Chronic skin conditions like eczema or psoriasis
- Diarrhea or constipation
- Fatigue
- Joint pain
- Mood imbalances like anxiety or depression
- Numbness of the hands or feet

NOTES FROM THE LAB

Some wheat breeders may seek to improve its taste and look by changing the gliadin-to-glutenin ratio. Unfortunately, such changes can introduce new peptides unfamiliar to the human digestive system. This can result in a leaky immune system, loss of oral tolerance, and the induction of non-celiac gluten sensitivity or possibly celiac disease.

lead to or exacerbate other debilitating autoimmune diseases, including type 1 diabetes, multiple sclerosis, gluten ataxia, inflammatory arthritis, psoriasis, and even neurodegenerative diseases such as Alzheimer's.

Researchers note that some gluten peptides can stimulate intestinal T cells in patients with celiac disease. In a recent study, celiac patients were screened for T cells against twenty-one different peptides in wheat. Predictably, they tested positive for gliadin and glutenin, but they also tested positive for several others. In a separate study, patients with non-celiac gluten sensitivity and Crohn's disease also reacted to an array of wheat proteins, not just the gliadin and glutenin. This shows that wheat challenges the immune system on several fronts.

12

DAIRY AND EGGS

Health is the result of living in harmony with yourself and the environment.

– Margo Adair, writer and activist

The origins of drinking the breast milk of another species have been debated for years. A 2019 analysis in *Archaeological and Anthropological Sciences* suggests it began 6,000 years ago with pastoral Neolithic Britons, evidenced by traces of dairy proteins found in calcified dental remains unearthed in three different archeological sites. The discovery has led scholars to speculate that these prehistoric people must have used processing methods—such as heating and fermenting—to reduce the lactose content, because, as it turns out, those first adventurous individuals were just as lactose intolerant and susceptible to the unpleasantries of dairy as 65 percent of the world population is today.

A curious thing happened to this early population of milk drinkers, however. Over the course of a millennia, a genetic mutation allowed them to digest fresh milk without the gut disturbances we typically associate with lactose intolerance. Known as lactase persistence, the trait is found in only about a third of the world's population, largely in European countries and to some degree (about 20 percent) in the United States. Lactase persisters also exist in small pockets of East Africa, the Middle East, and South Asia.

No one is born lactose intolerant—all mammals are born with the ability to digest lactose. Lactose is a disaccharide, a class of sugar that has two individual sugar molecules—glucose and galactose—linked together into one molecule. Our bodies can only absorb single sugar molecules, so we need to produce an enzyme called lactase to split the lactose molecule into individual sugars. Without lactase, we would not be able to digest the breast milk from our mothers.

As noted in Chapter 2, breastfeeding plays a big part in activating our adaptive immunity, creating our gut microbiome, and providing nutritional needs, including calcium, vitamin D, protein, vitamin B12, vitamin A, riboflavin, potassium, and phosphorus. Breast milk also contains probiotics and prebiotics—it's how the mother passes her immune protection to her baby until it can develop its immune system. For the very young, mother's milk is life-giving and easy to digest, but as mammals mature and are weaned, their bodies stop producing lactase because it's no longer needed. Still, many people in industrialized countries consume cow's milk long into adulthood. This presents a problem, since milk contains proteins that vary from mammal to mammal according to the nutritional needs of its species. In other words, human milk is the most beneficial nutrient for human infants, cow's milk is the most beneficial nutrient for calves, sheep's milk for lambs, and so on.

Cow's milk contains more than twenty proteins known to cause severe allergic reactions in humans. Nearly 10 percent of the U.S. population has a classic immunoglobulin E-mediated allergic reaction. There is also increasing awareness that children who consume cow's milk too early in life may be at risk for autoimmune conditions such as type 1 diabetes, celiac disease, Crohn's disease, Behçet's disease (an autoimmune disease of the blood vessels, skin, and mucus membranes. Common symptons are mouth sores, eye irritation, and skin rashes.), multiple sclerosis, or mild rheumatoid arthritis later in life. The American Academy of Pediatrics strongly recommends waiting until babies are at least a year old before introducing dairy products to their diets.

DAIRY AND AUTOIMMUNITY

Cow's milk contains twenty-five different proteins, with about 95 percent of them falling into two categories: caseins and whey. Casein comprises 80 percent of milk's proteins and is made up of four major components: alpha, beta, kappa, and gamma. Whey consists of beta-lactoglobulin, alpha-lactalbumin, immunoglobulins, and lactoferrin. During the digestive process, the body breaks down the milk proteins into peptides to make them easier for the small intestine to absorb, but the resulting amino acids can mimic collagen or cell antigens that induce disorders. Here's a further breakdown of dairy-related immune reactivity.

Granulocyte-macrophage colony-stimulating factor (GM-CSF). The mammary gland is the main site for expression of casein, but studies have looked at whether casein can be found in white blood cells, as they also express the alpha-casein gene. This matters because the addition of alpha-casein to these cells results in the production of granulocyte-macrophage colony-stimulating factor. This in turn stimulates innate and adaptive immune responses and plays a significant role in the development of autoimmune diseases.

The A1/A2 hypothesis. A controversial multi-country study out of New Zealand posits that a beta-casein may be responsible for a rise in certain autoimmune disorders. The theory goes that beta-casein comes in two forms: A1 and A2. A1 is suggested to be a driver behind type 1 diabetes, heart disease, schizophrenia, and autism. A2, on the other hand, appears to be neutral. A single cow can express both genotypic variations in her milk. In a 2018 peer-reviewed scientific paper my father and I co-authored, we showed that both A1 and A2 milks are immunologically identical, meaning that if a person reacts to one, they will equally react to the other.

Some individuals with autism improve when they switch to a casein- and gluten-free diet, possibly due to a changing microbiome, which helps heal a leaky gut and reduces the cross-reactive attack of the milk antibodies against neurological tissue.

BCM-7 peptides. Milk contains a peptide with opioid characteristics. Called beta-casomorphin-7 (BCM-7), this peptide has also been detected in the urine and blood samples of patients with neurological disorders. It can cause changes in the digestive tract, immune function, and brain development.

Some studies have suggested that BCM-7 may cause a range of chronic conditions, including type 1 diabetes, ischemic heart disease, autism, and schizophrenia. This peptide is also associated with stomach ulcers, ulcerative colitis, Crohn's disease, and celiac disease. The strongest evidence so far is for type I diabetes and heart disease.

Myelin basic protein (MBP) and myelin oligodendrocyte glycoprotein (MOG). In 2013, my father and I tested 400 people for milk reactivity. Our study demonstrated that up to 20 percent of those samples expressed immune reactivity to milk. About half also showed reactivity to major nerve cell antigens in the body, namely myelin basic protein (MBP) and myelin oligodendrocyte glycoprotein (MOG). MBP is a foundational protein of the nervous system, contributing to the outer-layer protection (referred to as a sheath) of nerve cells. MOG is a glycoprotein in the central nervous system. Both MBP and MOG are linked to multiple sclerosis and other immune disorders.

In another study, we determined that all varieties of cow's milk—organic, grass-fed, pasteurized, bottled, or otherwise—were unsuitable for susceptible individuals because they contained the same reactive proteins. Goat and sheep milk were 93 percent antigenically similar to cow's milk, while camel's milk proved very promising, as it had different beta-caseins, no beta-lactoglobulin, and very low immunoglobulins. Our overall results showed that the safest alternatives to cow's milk are—in descending order—human, camel, sheep, and goat milks.

EGGS AND AUTOIMMUNITY

When it comes to food-related autoimmunity, people tend to react in themes. For instance, many people who are sensitive to gluten are also sensitive to dairy, and those sensitive to dairy frequently have issues with eggs. All three food groups share similar protein sequences, which might explain lingering food reactivity even with a strict gluten-free diet because of unaddressed dairy and egg sensitivities.

Case in point: Chicken eggs contain forty-seven proteins, including a small-molecule enzyme called lysozyme, found in high concentrations in the egg white. Lysozyme is also found in human tears, saliva, milk, and mucous membranes as part of our innate immune system, and functions to attack invading bacterial cell walls. In egg whites, lysozyme protects the embryo chick from pathogens as it grows inside its porous eggshell.

Lysozyme, however, can be troublesome for anyone struggling with chronic viral infections or gut and autoimmune disorders, likely because lysozyme slips into the tight junctions of the gut lining and opens the gut barrier to other unwelcome proteins where they can access the bloodstream. Research also shows that egg

NOTES FROM THE LAB

Visit any coffee shop these days and you'll find cappuccinos available with non-dairy milk products. Grocery stores now offer scores of "milks" ranging from almond, macadamia, cashew, and hemp seed to oat, soy, and coconut. Like gluten-free products, you'll also see an impressive array of dairy-free substitutions, including almond-based ice creams, cashew cheese, and my personal favorite, coconut coffee creamer.

In 2018, my father and I conducted a study where we applied concentrations of animal milk protein and alternative milk proteins to the wells of a testing plate. Milk-specific IgE, IgG, and IgA antibodies were measured against goat, sheep, camel, and human milks, along with soy-, almond- and coconut-based milk substitutes in twenty-four blood samples that tested positive against cow's milk proteins.

Overall, coconut-based milk substitute was found to be the least allergenic and antigenic when compared to soy and almond milk. The takeaway from this is not to assume that plant milk substitutes are automatically a safer alternative to mammalian milks but to figure out what is safe for you and your body. Accurate testing of IgE, IgG, and IgA antibodies against different milks and plant-based substitutes can help you determine this.

whites cross-react with the Epstein-Barr virus.

In the lab, we tested yolks and whites separately and found both show reactivity. We also discovered that eggs can be a trigger for people with obsessive-compulsive disorder and Alzheimer's, and may be involved in irritable bowel syndrome, inflammatory bowel disease, Crohn's, ulcerative colitis, autoimmune thyroid disease, multiple sclerosis, neuromyelitis optica, and type 1.5 diabetes (a delayed-onset of type 1 diabetes). For this reason, I tell all my patients to avoid chicken eggs. Proteins structures in duck and quail eggs differ from chicken eggs, so most people tend to tolerate them much better.

13

LECTINS AND AQUAPORINS

An ounce of prevention is worth a pound of cure.

– Benjamin Franklin

Despite their lack of a brain or central nervous system, plants care more about their own survival than ours. Throughout their 700 million years of existence, plants have evolved to include some pretty ingenious defense systems: bark that discourages munching herbivores, secretions that attract the predators (hornets) of their predators (caterpillars), thorns and prickly spines that discourage touching, sap that traps insects, and poisons that sicken or kill when ingested. Lectins are one such poison.

Dubbed Mother Nature's pesticide, lectins are found in varying degrees in just about every living thing, from microorganisms to animals. They are most prevalent, however, in the seeds, skins, roots, and leaves of certain plants. These plants use lectin as a defense mechanism against intruders like insects, parasites, pathogens, molds, fungi, and foraging animals, including humans. When lectins are ingested, they can make predators feel sick, potentially deterring future indulgences.

Some lectins are safe for humans, while others, such as ricin derived from castor seeds, are downright deadly. Approximately 30 percent of our food contains lectins, including corn, wheat, peanuts, kidney beans, peas, lentils, soybeans, mushrooms, and rice. The greatest concentrations, however, are found in raw beans and grains (especially wheat), followed by commercial dairy products and plants in the nightshade family: tomatoes, tomatillos, goji berries, potatoes, eggplant, and all peppers. (Black pepper, incidentally, does not fall into this category.)

Reactions to lectins vary wildly. Some people can eat these foods with zero or mild effects, especially since soaking, sprouting, and cooking help break down some of the lectins. Enzymes produced during digestion also help degrade lectins, but they can be notoriously resistant. For many, particularly those with a compromised immune system, lectins can cause inflammation and increase gut permeability.

WAYS TO REDUCE LECTINS IN FOOD

I don't recommend consuming lectin-heavy foods if your gut is in an unhealthy state. Once your digestion normalizes, however, you may consider experimenting to see if you can eat them without issue. Some nutrition experts suggest that as long as lectins are deactivated by adequate soaking, sprouting, cooking, deseeding, or fermenting, the nutritive benefits outweigh their potential negative effects. Moreover, lectins exist primarily in the raw forms of foods, and usually in peels and seeds. This includes nuts (seeds of trees), grains (seeds of grasses), and legumes (seeds of flowering plants).

Still, the key is moderation. Some grains—wheat, oats, rye, barley, and spelt—should remain on your list of foods to permanently avoid, as noted in previous chapters. Additionally, no amount of processing can fully or even mostly remove the lectins in these foods. Here are some of the ways to remove excess lectin from the foods you consume.

Soaking nuts in water. The denser the nut, the longer the soak. Almonds, hazelnuts, and pistachios should soak for four to eight hours. Nuts with more oil, such as walnuts, pecans, and Brazil nuts, require less time, between two to four hours. Cashews, pine nuts, and macadamias require only about an hour. If some nuts float to the top, simply remove them. After soaking, lay them on paper towels and pat dry. Allow to thoroughly dry (preferably in sunlight or at 150 degrees Fahrenheit in the oven) before storing in an airtight glass container.

Sprouting involves soaking seeds and then allowing them to sprout. Through sprouting, the protective coating that allows seeds to stay dormant is removed, taking with it many of the lectins.

In the digestive tract, lectins bind to carbohydrates, but if there are too many, it can encourage abnormal colonization by harmful bacteria and protozoa. What's more, lectins tend to coagulate, or clump cells together, in a process known as agglutination (literally meaning to glue or cement in Latin). The result is inflammation, gas, and bloating.

After repeated consumption, dietary lectins induce the release of endotoxins such as lipopolysaccharides. As noted in previous chapters, the presence of lipopolysaccharides increases gut permeability and allows the passage of unwelcome particles—including sticky lectin molecules—into the bloodstream. Once in the circulation, lectins bind with other tissues that have lectin-like receptors, including connective tissue, thyroid, liver, and pancreas. Here's a short list of other places lectins tend to latch onto:

T cells, which may drive inflammation in joints and lead to rheumatoid arthritis.

Pancreas islet cells (where insulin is produced), which can lead to type 1 diabetes.

Glomerular basement membrane, a protein in the filtration system of the kidneys. The resulting autoimmune response causes glomerulonephritis, an acute inflammatory response in the kidney.

Human endometrium, spermatozoa, and ova, resulting in an autoimmune reaction that can cause infertility in men or women.

Because of their binding properties, lectins can also cause nutrient deficiencies, disrupt digestion, and cause severe intestinal damage when consumed in excess by anyone with dysfunctional enzymes or ongoing digestive issues. If you have heartburn, acid reflux, or any other digestive problem, consider removing lectin-rich foods from your diet to gauge your level of reactivity. As for lab work, Cyrex's Array 3 and Array 10 can zero in on specific triggers to help identify which ones to remove.

AQUAPORINS

The majority of cells in our bodies contain up to 60 percent water. Like breathing, we rarely think about the constant flow of water silently moving in and out of our cells, diligently removing waste, regulating our body temperature, lubricating our joints, and protecting our tissues. The mechanism within each cell that allows this constant transport of water is called an aquaporin. Also called "water channels," aquaporins are proteins with six spiraled channels that selectively allow water to enter and exit the cell.

Aquaporins also exist in plants—many that we eat, including spinach, soy, corn, and tomatoes. Since some of these aquaporin-rich foods are structurally similar to our own aquaporins, they can trace a path to autoimmunity through molecular mimicry, typically affecting aquaporin-4 (AQP4), found in the brain, central nervous system, lung, thyroid, stomach, and skeletal muscle. In the brain, AQP4 is believed to play a role in maintaining homeostasis and water exchange, electrical activity, and how nerves transmit information.

In 2015, my father and three of his colleagues published research that looked into molecular mimicry in the brain from aquaporin proteins, specifically in patients with multiple sclerosis (MS) and neuromyelitis optica (NMO), a central nervous system disorder that primarily affects eye nerves. Together, the team of scientists discovered a high correlation in antibody reaction between plant aquaporins and brain antigens and concluded that a subclass of patients with multiple sclerosis and neuromyelitis optica reacts to both plant and human AQP4 peptides. As an aside, neuromyelitis optica is more commonly found in Asian countries, and it's speculated that this phenomenon occurs due to the increased consumption of soybean and spinach by these populations.

Additional studies have implicated aquaporins in other neurological disorders, including Alzheimer's, autism, depression, and Parkinson's. In yet another study in which my father participated, 577 patients were assessed for food and neuronal tissue reactivity. Nearly 24 percent tested positive for at least one dietary aquaporin. The most reactive food containing aquaporin reactivity was spinach (79 percent), followed by corn (64 percent), tomato (37 percent), and soybean (26 percent). The study also revealed that women were slightly more susceptible than men.

Unfortunately, aquaporins are resilient and can survive food preparation and high temperatures. If you are unable to test your susceptibility to aquaporins, the following list of risk factors can serve as a guide. Avoid aquaporins if you have a history of:
- Leaky gut syndrome
- Rheumatoid arthritis

Deseeding tomatoes is easy as 1-2-3. First, place your tomatoes in a pot of water and bring to a boil for about five minutes before transferring to an ice bath. Second, once cooled, the skins, which also contain lectins, should peel away effortlessly. And third, cut the tomatoes in half and scoop out the seeds. Be aware, however, that tomatoes also contain aquaporins, so if you have reason to be concerned about neuroautoimmunity, consider limiting your consumption to special occasions or avoid altogether.

Heating is another good way to lower the lectin load. Beans are best deactivated by first bringing them to a boil, then allowing them to soak in the boiled water between eight to sixteen hours. After soaking, discard the water and simmer in fresh water at a high temperature (at least 203 degrees Fahrenheit) for an hour. I don't recommend slow cooking, especially for kidney beans (which are highly toxic in their raw form), as the water may not get hot enough to deactivate the lectins. Discard any beans that remain hard, as lectins may not be adequately destroyed.

Fermenting also breaks down lectins. While soybeans carry a heavy lectin load, fermented soy products like miso, tempeh, and natto are well tolerated.

- Frequent use of antibiotics
- A diet high in grains and legumes
- Family history of autoimmune disorders
- Mental health problems

NOTES FROM THE LAB

There are only four food aquaporins to look out for, ranked in order of most to least reactive:

- Spinach (79 percent)
- Corn (64 percent)
- Tomato (37 percent)
- Soybean (26 percent)

According to Steven Gundry, MD, author of the acclaimed book *The Plant Paradox*, which takes a deep dive into the world of lectins, the following list highlights the foods containing the highest levels of lectin:

- Conventionally raised meat (corn is usually fed to the animals)
- Corn
- Cereal grains
- Legumes and beans (including peanuts)
- Nightshade fruits and vegetables (tomatoes, tomatillos, eggplant, goji berries, all peppers, white potatoes, and red spices such as paprika, curry, chili powder, and cayenne)
- Quinoa
- Vegetable oils made with corn, soy, and sunflower oil

While Dr. Gundry advocates universal adoption of a lectin-free diet, I tend to be much more flexible in this area. In 2018, my father and I conducted research showing that only individuals with specific immune reactivity—particularly those living with rheumatoid arthritis and a positive rheumatoid factor to lectins—should follow this very challenging elimination. That said, reducing lectin content in food can be a useful and helpful dietary intervention for all.

SIGNS OF LECTIN AND AQUAPORIN REACTIVITY

- Bloating, gas, and abdominal cramps
- Painful and swollen joints
- Watery eyes, runny nose, and congestion
- Fatigue and tiredness
- Depression
- Hormonal fluctuations
- Nausea after meals
- Skin rashes

14

SUGAR, SALT, AND ADDITIVES

You never fail until you stop trying.

– Albert Einstein

Food used to be simple. It grew or lived off the earth, you killed it or picked it off a plant, and then you ate it. No middleman, no baggage. Then we figured out how to save food for later. We preserved meats and fish with salt, and somewhere during that process, people realized that salt marvelously enhanced flavor and made each bite more savory. Mankind later discovered that adding sugar to fruit preserved it in the form of delicious seasonal jams. If not for the advent of sanitation and modern medicine that allowed humans to live longer, we might have never fully realized that excessive amounts of salt and sugar can do a person in by middle age, like cause gallstones, kidney stones, rising blood pressure, and cardiovascular disease.

As the world evolved over the centuries, so did our relationship with food. Rather than eating solely to survive, we began eating and snacking for pleasure. We also started consuming meals on the go, because who has time to raise and grow their own food, much less prepare it these days? This is how sugar, salt, and additives took hold in our modern diet.

You can see it for yourself as you cruise the aisles of the local grocery store. Grab a bag of cheese-dusted corn chips off the shelf. Most likely, the corn used to make this crunchy snack is genetically modified and grown in a field sprayed with pesticides. Once it's harvested, it's shipped off to a factory to be processed into a corn chip. Salt and preservatives are added to give the chip more flavor and the ability to sit on a shelf for months or years. Next, it gets deep fried in industrialized vegetable oil. After that, the chip is dusted with a mix of artificial ingredients that sort of taste like cheese. Then a food dye is added so your eyes are tricked into thinking you're eating something made with real cheese. And finally, after the rigorous process from field to factory to artificially cheesy snack, a handful of chips are dropped into a crinkly bag teeming with chemicals and toxins.

By the time you grab the bag and rip it open for your snacking pleasure, the chips are so far removed from nature that it's surprising it can even be labeled "food." With each one of those crunchy chips, you introduce your body to an array of substances that can cause inflammatory responses. Yet you dive in with excitement and finish by licking each finger clean to enjoy that last bit of "cheese" dust.

In this chapter, we'll look at some of the additives that make our foods more colorful, flavorful, and desirable, and far less nutritious—like sugar, artificial sweeteners, table salt, colorings, gums, and meat glue. (Yes, meat glue!) We'll also look at some of the indirect additives that make it into our food supply by way of pesticides, plastics, and more.

THE NOT-SO-SWEET TRUTH ON ADDED SUGAR AND ARTIFICIAL SWEETENERS

We can divide sugar into two camps: naturally occurring and added. The former is found in only two types of foods: lactose in milk and fructose in fruit. The latter is found in honey, maple syrup, molasses, malt sugar, brown sugar, white sugar, agave syrup, high-fructose corn syrup, and anything ending in the suffix "ose," like dextrose, maltose, and sucrose. We call these "added" sugars because we don't sit down and eat them by themselves but add them to other foods such as coffee, tea, sodas, cereals, desserts, condiments, sauces, salad dressings, crackers, flavored yogurts, and breads. The list is almost endless.

Scientifically speaking, sugar is a sweet, short-chain, soluble carbohydrate. The type most people know and use as table or granulated sugar is sucrose, which the body converts into fructose and glucose. More complex long-chain sugars are called oligosaccharides. It used to be that any kind of sugar was a rare thing. In prehistoric times, people in New Guinea chewed on reeds to derive their sweetness. Then sugarcane made its way to India through trade routes. It wasn't until around 2,000 years ago, in about 5 AD, that people in India began evaporating cane juice into crystals, which made transportation to other countries much easier. (The word "sugar" comes from the Sanskrit word sarkara. Likewise, we get the word "candy" from the Indian word khanda, or sugar crystals.) At any rate, sugar was, until relatively recent times, a rare luxury, enjoyed exclusively by the very rich.

The bad news is that added sugars are, well, really bad news. They contain no essential nutrients. They rot your teeth. They can disrupt your body's ability to produce insulin. In short, added sugars put you at risk for obesity, diabetes, cancer, and liver disease. So why do we love sugar so much? Because it tastes good and feels good, and when we eat it, it causes the reward center of the brain to release massive amounts of the feel-good chemical dopamine, potentially creating a sugar addiction.

Unfortunately, that's not all. Combining sugar with proteins and heat (like on a barbecue), creates advanced glycation end products (AGEs), also known as glycotoxins, compounds that show significance in the development of diabetes and other chronic diseases. AGEs are a part of normal metabolism, but when levels in tissues and the circulatory system are excessively high, they can become pathogenic, or cause disease. AGEs also cross-react with body proteins and alter their structure and function.

AGEs and their receptor (RAGE) have also been linked to diabetic vascular disease, osteoarthritis, cellular dysfunction, and cancer. What's more, antibodies against cooked food antigens react with AGEs and tissue proteins, potentially resulting in atherosclerosis, neurodegeneration, and neuroautoimmunity.

Many people trying to avoid sugar's negative effects instead turn to artificial sweeteners like aspartame (NutraSweet, Equal), saccharin (Sweet'N Low, Sugar Twin), sucralose (Splenda), and acesulfame potassium (Sweet One, Swiss Sweet, Sunett). Ongoing research suggests that theses sweeteners disrupt the gut-brain axis by changing the composition of the intestinal microbiome.

Then there are natural, plant-based sugar substitutes like stevia, mangosteen extract, and allulose. Emerging research suggests that stevia can disrupt hormones and exacerbate thyroid conditions, though it seems to be a bigger problem with daily use longer than six months rather than with occasional use. Mangosteen extract and allulose are also somewhat worrisome, but there's currently no research to back it up. One of the latest sweeteners circulating among the health conscious is monk fruit extract. So far, most news has been positive—it's safe for diabetics and doesn't spike blood sugar, and some say it's even anti-inflammatory. Still, a small percentage of people have reported allergic reactions, so like all sweeteners, it's best to indulge in moderation.

As for agave syrup—formally the darling of the health conscious—it's problematic as well. It falls in the so-called natural category and doesn't spike blood sugar, but it is predominately pure fructose (without the fiber), and recent research suggests that it promotes obesity and contributes to type 2 diabetes. For those reasons, I can no longer support the use of agave syrup as a healthful alternative.

Sugar alcohols like xylitol, erythritol, and sorbitol have become especially alluring in recent years. They are low glycemic, won't spike blood sugar, contain half the calories of sugar, and taste pretty darn good. They're also derived from plant-based sources, so they're not artificial in the same way as aspartame. Sounds great, right? Not so fast. Sugar alcohols are a type of carbohydrate often derived from genetically modified corn sugar and corn starch. Even xylitol, which is sometimes derived from a non-genetically modified source like the birch tree, is problematic because it has undergone a process known as sugar hydrogenation, which rearranges the structure of the fructose molecule.

It's important to note that all sugar alcohols are highly, highly processed. This results in a low-digestible carbohydrate that disrupts the gut and triggers gas, bloating, and diarrhea. Over time, the extended use of sugar alcohols can contribute to gut dysbiosis.

My suggestion is to use natural sweeteners like stevia very sparingly as a rare treat rather than part of your everyday lifestyle. Even better, stick with tried-and-true sweeteners found in honey, 100 percent maple syrup, molasses, coconut sugar, and now monk fruit extract—but again, use them sparingly and in moderation.

EASY ON THE SALT

Next to fire, salt may be the greatest thing in history to impact the science of cooking. It's no wonder that saltiness is one of the basic human tastes, since the human body is made up of about 1 percent sodium—found abundantly in our blood, sweat, and tears. Salt adds zing and savor to food and kicks it up a notch. Our natural affinity for it is also shared by other animals, who show their love for it by flocking to salt licks.

Unlike other additives, salt actually serves a vital purpose in our bodies. It helps nerves and muscles function properly and is one of the factors involved in maintaining the body's fluid balance. When athletes strain their bodies, they must rehydrate to restore their water and mineral levels. Salt was so precious in ancient times, in fact, that it was literally worth its weight in gold. That's where the word "salary" comes from—it's the Latin word for salt because the Roman legions were paid with it. It's also where we get the saying that someone is "worth his salt." In the days of yore, if you ate a man's salt at his table, you were obliged not to harm him.

The problem is that we overdo it. The habitual salt intake in Western countries is generally higher than in Eastern Europe and Asia. In the United States, land of fast food, 77 percent of the sodium eaten comes from processed and restaurant food.

High salt consumption is associated with a greater risk of stroke and cardiovascular disease. Insufficient water intake, obesity, high cholesterol, and other factors can also lead to the accumulation of salt and other minerals within the organs, producing gallstones and kidney stones. Nearly nine in ten children eat more salt than recommended, and about one in six children (yes, children) have elevated blood pressure, placing them at massively increased risk for stroke and heart disease in adulthood.

Salt is also associated with autoimmune disease. Studies show that too much dietary salt increases the production of pro-inflammatory T-helper 17 cells in the gut, which in turn increases the development of symptoms consistent with multiple sclerosis. Even a modest increase in salt contributes to inflammation, neuroexcitability, cell proliferation, and cell death. One study with mice shows a link between high salt intake and problems with memory and learning.

So, yes, salt is tasty, useful, and necessary for our bodies to sustain life, but like any good thing, too much of it can be bad.

A DISTURBING RAINBOW OF ARTIFICIAL FOOD COLORS

If you knew a chemical had the capacity to bind to your DNA and damage it, would you want it in your food? Of course not. If you're purchasing packaged foods, chances are that you've been eating them just the same. They come in the form of Blue 1, Blue 2, Citrus Red 2, Green 3, Orange B, Red 3, Red 40, Yellow 5, Yellow 6, and more. Artificial food dyes are so ubiquitous that we rarely notice them anymore. They're in caramel-colored lattes, microwave popcorn, flavored yogurts, energy bars, bottled salad dressings, farm-raised salmon, and even pickles and tandoori chicken.

Additionally, just about any food geared toward children is laden with artificial food coloring: candies, cereals, chewing gum, sodas, juices, chips and crackers, fruit leathers, frozen foods, macaroni and cheese, and, of course, rainbow-sprinkled cakes, cupcakes, and other desserts.

Artificial coloring is also added to medicines, mouthwash, toothpastes, soaps, lotions, and creams, and it can be absorbed orally or through the skin. These colorings are often added for no other reason than visual appeal. But at what cost? Over the past fifty years, manufacturers have increased their use by 500 percent. During that same time, we've witnessed an alarming rise in childhood behavioral problems such as aggression, allergies, attention deficit disorder (ADD), and attention deficit/hyperactivity disorder (ADHD), which now affects 11 percent of children. These additives are unhealthy for everyone because they change the composition of our foods and can also alter our DNA in ways that confuse and provoke the immune system.

For starters, artificial food dyes are made from petroleum, also known as crude oil—the same stuff in gasoline. The food and pharmaceutical industries prefer petroleum-derived synthetic food colorants over natural ones because they are cheaper, more easily available, and longer lasting, and can achieve those unnatural neon hues kids love.

Food manufacturers like artificial colorings because they bind so readily with food proteins. Unfortunately, they also bind quite easily with proteins in the human body. Have you ever seen a child's tongue and lips turn a bright color from eating a snow cone or cotton candy? That's from the artificial dye binding to human tissue. One autopsy study showed an entire colon dyed bright green from food coloring.

Studies on dogs and rats found that while most food dyes are excreted through feces and urine, significant amounts remain adhered to the intestinal walls. This indicates that dyes or their metabolites can bind to human tissue and form new compounds foreign to the immune system. Repeated use of foods, cosmetics, or drugs containing artificial colors can accumulate in your body tissue, creating new antigens for the immune system to attack, which leads to autoimmune reactivity.

Once the dye binds with human tissue, it presents the immune system with a confusing new compound. This is one way autoimmunity develops. Unfortunately, this scenario often plays out in the brain, too, and could explain the connection between food dyes and neurobehavioral issues in children and adults.

Other conditions linked to food coloring include allergic rhinitis, asthma, chronic hives, welts, runny nose, atopic dermatitis, angioedema, and liver disease. Additionally, people with salicylate sensitivity cannot tolerate aspirin or Yellow No. 5, which can cause asthma and hives. Yellow 5 is often present in soft drinks, energy drinks, gummy bears, marshmallow treats, cotton candy, cookies, jams and jellies, cereals, noodles, dill sauce, pickles, and more. It's also in crayons, cleaning products, and envelope glues.

Food manufacturers aren't required to list the amount of food dye in their products, and in 2010, the FDA raised the permitted amount of food dye per person from 12 mg per day (established in 1950) to 62 mg. The amount found to cause behavioral issues in children is 30 mg. That's less than what is found in a single bowl of colorful cereal, a single-serving package of colorful candy, or an artificially colored beverage.

Many children today easily consume 100 to 200 mg a day of artificial food colorings.

The research on food dyes prompted the European Union to require warning labels on foods with dyes, but none are required in the United States. Still, some manufacturers are voluntarily removing them from their products amid growing concern. It's always a good idea to read labels carefully and stick with dye-free foods.

PROBLEMATIC FOOD GUMS

The word "gum" probably evokes blowing bubbles and trading baseball cards, but gums actually play a large role in the food industry. Employed as stabilizers, emulsifiers, and thickening, gelling, and fixing agents, gums are everywhere—in soups, ice cream, soft drinks, cakes, pies, jellies, candies, yogurts, vegan nut milks, gluten-free pastas, and more. In 1993 alone, the world market for gums as food additives was about $10 billion U.S., not including non-food uses for gums. While the FDA labels them "generally recognized as safe," gums are linked to food immune and allergic reactions. What's more, studies have shown that gums are structurally similar to a number of common foods, so cross-reactivity is possible.

Since 1933, when a case of asthma caused by acacia gum came to light, work-related incidents involving the inhalation of gums have received a decent amount of attention. In simple terms, gums in the lungs are a bad thing. We studied how gums react in the gut, and 288 healthy subjects found significant immune reactivity against various gum extracts. For example, an immunoglobulin G response against gum tragacanth was found in 5.2 percent of the tested individuals, and against carrageenan in 27 percent. The results of our study show that a subgroup of healthy subjects who produce immunoglobulin G and immunoglobulin E antibodies against various gums may suffer from hidden food immune reactivities and sensitivities. Some studies indicate that patients allergic to pollen can also experience immune reactivity to gum.

Gums degrade the quality of whole foods, and ample evidence suggests they can cause gastrointestinal distress, bloating, abdominal gas, and loose stools in sensitive individuals. People with leaky gut, digestive issues, autoimmune disorders, and pollen allergies might want to severely limit or remove gums entirely from their diet. Listed here are some of the most widely used gums you'll find on food labels.

Carob gum (locust bean gum) starts as a whitish powder obtained from grinding the endosperm of the seeds of *Ceratonia siliqua*, a tree widely cultivated in the Mediterranean region. Carob gum is used in products including ice cream, baby foods, soups, sausage products, soft cheeses and other dairy items, bakery goods, pie fillings, powdered desserts, sauces, salad, creams, and pet foods. Carob gum is known to cause gas in some people.

Carrageenan is extracted from various red algae and used for thickening and stabilizing dairy products, imitation creams, puddings, syrups, and canned pet foods. It is also used in the manufacture of shampoos, cosmetics, shoe polish, and medicines. Because it is sourced from a plant, carrageenan is often found in products marked vegan and all-natural. That said, several studies suggest that carrageenan triggers inflammation and gastrointestinal ulcers. In animal studies, carrageenan has been shown to induce tumors and ulcers.

Gellan gum is fermented from plants by bacteria. In animal studies, it has been shown to disrupt the lining of the digestive tract.

Guar gum comes from the Indian legume *Cyamopsis tetragonoloba*; it is primarily the ground endosperm of guar beans. In some people, guar gum causes gas, bloating, and loose stools.

Gum arabic (acacia gum) is the oldest and best known of all-natural gums. It derives its name from its place of origin, ancient Egypt, where it was used as a binder and adhesive for pigments, paints, inks, cosmetics, and flaxen wrappings for mummies. Gum arabic comes from the stems and branches of Acacia senegal or Acacia seyal plants. This gum seems to be tolerable for most people.

Xanthan, like gellan gum, is fermented from plants (typically corn, soy, or wheat) by bacteria (from dairy) and is found in many gluten-free foods. In large amounts, xanthan has a laxative effect and can cause gas and diarrhea. Because it has also been shown to increase the frequency of bacterial infection and intestinal inflammation in infants, the FDA has banned it from use in infant formulas.

TRANSGLUTAMINASE, OR 'MEAT GLUE'

Meat glue exists, and it does exactly what its name implies: It glues chunks of meat or other foods together. Meat glue has been banned in the European Union since 2010, but its production is going strong in the United States and other parts of the world.

Known scientifically as transglutaminase, meat glue is made by cultivating the bacteria found in the blood of pigs and cows. (Transglutaminase is also found in various tissues throughout the human body and helps blood form clots.) Transglutaminase is often mixed in with gelatin and a milk derivative called caseinate, and maltodextrin, powdered skim milk, anti-caking agents, and trisodium phosphate can also be added.

Transglutaminase is actually a ubiquitous enzyme, present in yeast, fungi, and many plants and microorganisms, particularly *Streptomyces mobaraensis*, a spore-forming bacterium. When purified from the *Streptomyces*, it's called microbial transglutaminase, mTG, or food glue. In powder form, microbial transglutaminase is used to shape fish without bones, to turn flakes of white fish into imitation crabmeat, and to mold chicken scraps into nuggets.

The troubling thing is that the food industry is not required to tell you whether it's in products. Transglutaminase is used to make tofu firmer, to provide texture in baked goods (particularly gluten-free varieties), and to thicken some milks, yogurts, and packaged egg whites. Likewise, it is used in some medications to make them more water-soluble, non-aggregating, non-immunogenic, and more stable against digestion. You won't find the term "meat glue" on labels, however. Instead, labels typically list maltodextrin and sodium caseinate along with transglutaminase.

Because of its unlimited use, the question is whether or not this enzyme increases the immunological properties of the proteins or peptides in our bodies. Studies have shown that continuous consumption of these industrially processed foods directly or indirectly may result in celiac disease, non-celiac gluten sensitivity, irritable bowel syndrome, and other autoimmunities.

The amounts of these potentially reactive substances contained in products should at least be disclosed on the labels. This is especially important for the subgroup of people who are more sensitive to these products.

ROUNDUP, BPA, AND ALUMINUM

Indirect additives are trace substances that leach into our foods during production, packaging, and storage. This includes harmful pesticides, aluminum, and bisphenol A, commonly known as BPA.

In 1974, Monsanto introduced the product Roundup to replace the banned synthetic insecticide dichlorodiphenyltrichloroethane, or DDT. Since then, Roundup, or glyphosate, and its cousin products have become the most widely used pesticide in the United States.

Today, glyphosate is quite literally everywhere—in the air, soil, water, and on our crops. (Crops do absorb pesticides and no amount of washing will fully get rid of them.) It's also in our meat and poultry, because the animals feed off grains dusted with Roundup. Even though glyphosate is strongly pushed by such giant food industry multinational companies as Monsanto and the Bayer Corporation, it is extremely toxic. It's even been labeled by the World Health Organization as "probably carcinogenic in humans."

Now, consider BPA, used in plastic bottles and the lining of some cans and papers. More than 90 percent of the population in the United States has a detectable level in their urine. BPA is absorbed by food if the package is compromised when exposed to heat (leaving plastic bottles in your car, microwaving Tupperware, and so on). Moreover, research has also found microplastics in fish.

The issue is that BPA and its substitutes are endocrine disruptors that bind to hormone receptors, such as estrogen, and disrupt their normal function. This can have significant potential impact on infants, children, and adults. With infertility and hormonal issues on the rise in the United States, I often ponder how much is linked to BPA exposure. Information is now emerging that BPA alternatives like bisphenol S (BPS) are causing alarming harm to brain cells.

Aluminum, while generally accepted as a great discovery of modern times, has demonstrated toxicity to the GI tract, musculoskeleton, and nervous system, often resulting in autoimmunities, according to studies in animals and humans. It's also a neurotoxin and is associated with Alzheimer's and Parkinson's disease. Research has also found traces of aluminum in the nucleus of the neuron cells located in the brain.

In addition to foil, aluminum is used as a thickener, stabilizer, or anti-caking and raising agent in many foods, including cake mixes, cheeses, baking powder, and more. We are now finding that 40 percent of the aluminum we ingest is absorbed into the epithelial cells of the gut. Once the gut is leaky, aluminum can make its way to the bloodstream and into the brain.

FINAL THOUGHTS

All the food additives we just touched on have the potential to wreak havoc on your immune system. Unfortunately, they are present in just about every aspect of civilization. Thanks to agriculture machinery, factory assembly lines, chemicals, pasteurization, sterilization, and other innovations, the Industrial Revolution helped eliminate famine and provide us with a broader range of inexpensive foods. But it also turned our food into consumer products, which means manufacturers are constantly looking for ways to increase profits. The goal is to make their food products tastier, prettier, cheaper, and able to endure a much longer shelf life than the traditional foods humans have enjoyed for thousands of years.

According to a 2015 report published by the Israel Institute of Technology, autoimmune diseases have steadily increased alongside the expansion of food additives. The report suggests that industrialized additives increase intestinal permeability by breaching the integrity of tight junctions. As discussed in previous chapters, tight junction dysfunction is common in multiple autoimmune diseases.

Navigating the modern food supply can be complicated, but you do have the power to intervene and help your immune system focus on its job by steering toward the right foods. We'll explore this more in the next section.

PART IV:
REPAIR THE BARRIER

15

EATING TO THRIVE

Every day, in every way, I am getting better and better.

– Émile Coué, French psychologist

Disease begins in the gut, and that's also where healing begins. In this chapter, we'll take a closer look at nutrient-rich foods that support your immune system and help repair your gut barrier and oral tolerance.

A host of delicious, nourishing foods await, and they contain the nutrients necessary to establish a diverse and abundant bacterial community in your gut, fight off inflammation in your body, and leave you feeling rejuvenated. The foods mentioned here also support healthy Treg cells and regulate tolerance toward friendly bacteria and food proteins by downregulating T-helper 1 and 17 cells, which play pivotal roles in autoimmune diseases.

Eating to thrive is not a diet but a mindset, a customized lifestyle geared toward your specific health needs, so be sure to use your own discretion and avoid any personal dietary triggers on this list. Common triggers are marked with an asterisk (*).

FRUITS AND VEGETABLES

At least half of your plate should be covered in plants, since fruits and vegetables contain natural anti-inflammatory compounds. They're also rich sources of fiber that help lower levels of C-reactive protein, a marker linked to rheumatoid arthritis and other inflammatory disorders. Dark leafy greens like kale, swiss chard, and watercress are loaded with magnesium, folate, and other B vitamins that work alongside tryptophan to produce serotonin, the feel-good transmitter that helps ward off depression.

Cruciferous vegetables in particular are nutritional powerhouses loaded with indole-3-carbinol that help stimulate detoxifying enzymes in the gut and liver. These enzymes break down large molecules into smaller ones that can safely travel throughout the body to create energy. They also combat bad bugs in the gut. What's more, cruciferous veggies are high in fiber and contain rich amounts of folate, vitamin K, and sulfur. Incidentally, sulfur is required to build and fix DNA and protect cells from damage. Darker cruciferous veggies also bring vitamins A and C and phytonutrients that help reduce inflammation.

Organic leafy greens include romaine lettuce, kale, mustard greens, *spinach, watercress, collard greens, beet greens, swiss chard, arugula, endive, and turnip greens.

Organic vegetables include anise, artichokes, asparagus, beets, bok choy, broccoli, cabbage, carrots, cauliflower, celery, chives, cucumbers, fennel root, garlic, kohlrabi, leeks, onions, parsley, radishes, rhubarb, seaweed, shallots, squash, sugar snap peas, sweet potatoes, water chestnuts, watercress, yams, and zucchini.

Organic cruciferous vegetables and sprouts include arugula, bok choy, broccoli, brussels sprouts, cabbage, cauliflower, collard greens, kale, mustard greens, radishes, red cabbage, swiss chard, and watercress. For those with irritable bowel syndrome, ulcerative colitis, or other chronic intestinal conditions, the sulfur content in cruciferous vegetables may present gas and bloating issues. In this case, it's best to consume the sprouts of cruciferous veggies, such as broccoli and radishes, which are much gentler and provide exceptional healing properties. Leafy cruciferous veggies are also well tolerated.

Organic fruits include blueberries, strawberries, raspberries, bananas, blackberries, cherries, apples, apricots, avocados, grapefruit, grapes, kiwi, lemon, limes, lychee, oranges, peaches, pears, pineapple, plantains, plums, and watermelon. With the exception of avocado, consume no more than one serving a day from the fruit category.

WILD-CAUGHT FISH AND FARM-RAISED BIVALVES

Cold-water fish such as wild-caught salmon, trout, mackerel, and herring are among the healthiest foods on the planet. Not only are these fish delicious but they're also loaded with omega-3 fatty acids that aid in reducing inflammation. Other nutrients include protein and tryptophan metabolites, which help maintain gut mucosal homeostasis.

Swordfish, most tuna, and king mackerel are very high in mercury, so limit or avoid these completely. Instead, select "clean fish" sourced from waters with low contaminant contact and avoid fish sourced in waters with oil spills and pollution. Also look out for farm-raised fish, which are contained in cramped areas (like pigs and cows) and often given antibiotics to survive any illness induced by overcrowded quarters. The exceptions are farm-raised mollusks such as clams, oysters, and mussels. Bivalves are fantastically nutritious, providing vitamin B12, selenium, magnesium, and omega-3 fatty acids.

Low-mercury fish is particularly beneficial to those with autoimmune arthritis and joint-related diseases. Several studies indicate it can relieve tender joints and ease morning stiffness. Strive for at least four servings a week to get the full benefits.

Fatty fish and seafood include anchovies, *clams, halibut, herring, mackerel, *mussels, *oysters, rainbow trout, salmon, sardines, *scallops, and *shrimp.

LEAN, FREE-RANGE, GRASS-FED, ORGANICALLY GROWN ANIMAL PROTEIN

Animal protein can be a healing, nutrient-dense food loaded with minerals and nutrients that help calm allergies and combat inflammation. For red meat, choose grass-fed only, as conventionally raised meat is inhumane and also causes inflammation. This is because factory-farmed animals are fed unnatural diets filled with wheat and GMO corn and soy, and then injected with hormones and antibiotics.

Conversely, grass-fed beef provides a number of health benefits. First, it's leaner and contains double the amount of omega-3s of conventionally raised beef. Second, it contains conjugated linoleic acid, a type of fatty acid that calms the immune system and decreases the risk of insulin resistance; vitamin B12, which helps with memory, strengthens the gut lining, and protects the fatty myelin sheaves on nerve endings; and choline, which aids memory, boosts metabolism, and protects the heart. Other nutrients include B6, phosphorus, selenium, iron, potassium, and riboflavin.

Organ meats such as chicken liver are also especially healing. One 100 g serving is loaded with vitamins A, B2, B3, B12, D, folate, zinc, and iron. Dietary vitamin A is particularly healing for both the skin and the gut lining. It also stabilizes the immune system.

Dietary tryptophan—found in turkey, chicken, beef, pork, fish, seeds, nuts, beans, and dark chocolate— also plays an important role in immune function.

Meats includes grass-feed beef, grass-fed bison, grass-fed lamb, wild boar, and *pasture-raised pork and nitrate-free bacon. Undercooked pork can transmit *Yersinia* bacteria and cause reactive arthritis and joint issues, so I generally tell my patients with these conditions to avoid pork altogether. If you choose to eat pork, make sure to select pasture-raised and without nitrates.

Poultry and eggs include wild or pasture-raised turkey, pasture-raised chicken, wild or pasture-raised duck, and wild or pasture-raised quail. Duck, quail, and geese eggs are fine, too.

Animal fat such as cultured ghee, with its reduced casein content, is fine to consume. However, lard, duck, and goose fat can exacerbate the release of lipopolysaccharides because of their high saturated fat content, so those are best to avoid.

Bone broth is made with chicken, turkey, pork, beef, or lamb bones. Make sure you get meaty bones with a high collagen content by choosing those with an abundance of connective tissue, such as feet, knuckles, and necks. If you prefer to purchase premade broth, brands I trust include Bonafide Provisions and Kettle & Fire. Loaded with minerals like calcium, magnesium, phosphorus, boron, potassium, manganese, and zinc; vitamins A, K, C, and the B's; and amino acids like arginine, glutamine, cysteine, and L-glutamine, bone broth nourishes your gut lining and provides relief for painful joints. Bone broth is especially healing for inflammatory gut conditions such as ulcerative colitis and celiac disease. Whether you purchase your broth or make it yourself, be sure the bones used are from grass-fed or pasture-raised animals.

MEDICINAL MUSHROOMS AND FUNGI

The healing power of mushrooms has been long established in Eastern medicine. Happily, Western medicine and the biopharmaceutical industry are starting to catch up. Mushrooms are increasingly used to treat a wide variety of diseases, and emerging research shows they may be effective at treating allergic asthma, food allergy, atopic dermatitis, inflammation, autoimmune joint inflammation, gastrointestinal tract diseases, and cancer. Mushrooms truly are immune supportive, so enjoy heartily.

Mushrooms and fungi include beech, black trumpet, button, chaga, chanterelle, cordyceps, cremini, hedgehog, king trumpet, lion's mane, lobster, maitake, matsutake, morel, oyster, porcini, portobello, reishi, shiitake, truffle, and turkey tail.

FERMENTED FOODS

Including probiotic-rich fermented vegetables in your diet is an excellent way to restore gut health. The good bacteria they provide helps you digest complex carbohydrates and better absorb nutrients, fight off bad bacteria, and balance the pH in your gut.

Fermented foods include apple cider vinegar, coconut yogurt or kefir (unsweetened), kimchi, kombucha tea, kvass, miso, pickles, pickled ginger, and sauerkraut.

GLUTEN-FREE GRAINS AND OTHER WHEAT ALTERNATIVES

Once you heal your gut, you might consider adding back gluten-free grains if you are not sensitive to them. This includes gluten-free bread, crackers, and noodles. Gluten-free sourdough bread makes a nice addition, as it also contains some healthy probiotics—just make sure it doesn't contain more than one gum, and preferably none. The Resources section at the back of this book includes the brands I prefer.

Gluten-free grains and other wheat alternatives include amaranth, arrowroot flour, brown rice, brown shirataki yam noodles, cassava noodles (brand name Jovial), coconut flour, gluten-free bread, quinoa, rice flour, rolled oats and steel-cut oats (gluten-free), sesame or plain rice crackers, teff flour, and tigernut flour.

LEGUMES

As discussed in Chapter 13, I don't recommend lectin-heavy foods if your gut is still healing. Once your digestion normalizes and you're sure legumes are not trigger foods for you, you can benefit from their healing properties. Be sure to soak your beans and cook them well before consuming.

*Legumes include black beans, chickpeas, great northern beans, green beans, lentils, snap peas, snow peas, and yellow split peas.

PLANT-BASED DAIRY ALTERNATIVES

Forget about the days of soy milk as your only non-dairy alternative to milk. Today, we have access to a world of non-dairy plant-based milks, many fortified with calcium and vitamin D. When selecting milk alternatives, always choose those labeled as unsweetened. Also, be sure to check the ingredients list and avoid any containing carrageenan, maltodextrose, polysorbate 80, or carboymethyl cellulose. Another alternative is to make your own.

I don't recommend milks made from soy, oat, pea, or rice. Soy and pea are legumes and may be difficult for some people to digest. Oat and rice are both high in carbohydrates and may raise blood sugar.

Plant-based diary alternatives include milk made from almonds, cashews, coconut, hemp seeds, and macadamia nuts. Products made by MALK and Forager Project contain no gums or added sugar. Check the Resources section in the back of the book for more information.

Non-dairy coconut products include coconut butter, coconut cream, coconut flour, coconut milk, coconut oil, unsweetened coconut flakes, and unsweetened coconut yogurt and kefir.

NUTS AND SEEDS

If you have no sensitivities to nuts or seeds, they can be incredibly nutritious in modest quantities. Choose raw nuts and be sure to soak and/or sprout them to remove most of the lectins.

Nuts and seeds in this category include almond butter, Brazil nuts, almonds, cashews, chia seeds, hemp seeds, ground flaxseeds, macadamia nuts, pecans, pistachios, poppy seeds, pumpkin seeds, roasted sesame seeds, sunflower seeds, tahini, and walnuts.

HERBS AND SPICES

Not only do herbs and spices add flavor to our food but because they come from plants, they're also packed with phytochemicals and all sorts of other nutritional goodness. Ginger aids with digestion, turmeric calms inflammation, sage can improve memory, fenugreek improves blood sugar, and cinnamon helps lower cholesterol and triglycerides. Look for spices and herbs that are non-irradiated. (Irradiating involves using ionized radiation to kill insects and increase shelf life.) Instead, buy fresh, high-quality, and organic. Alternatively, you can grow your own herb garden and pick as needed.

Herbs and spices include allspice*, basil, bay leaf, black pepper, chili powder*, chives, cilantro, cinnamon*, coriander, cumin*, curry powder*, dill, fenugreek, garlic powder, ginger, leek, lemongrass, mint, mustard, onion powder, oregano, parsley, rosemary, sage, sea salt, thyme, and turmeric.

PLANT-BASED FATS

Monounsaturated fats are a major component in brain cells and contain anti-inflammatory properties that may work as effectively as aspirin or ibuprofen. What's more, olive oil contains a compound called oleocanthal that blocks inflammation-causing enzymes and decreases joint pain by 25 percent. A study conducted at Temple University in 2019 found that compounds in extra-virgin olive oil reduce the brain changes that lead to Alzheimer's disease.

In recent years, we've seen the arrival of avocado oil and MCT oil (derived from coconuts). Both are great flavor-neutral oils for dressings, but for cooking, avocado oil is best, with a smoke point of 500 degrees. It's worth noting that refined, polyunsaturated oils like canola, corn, soybean, and safflower easily go rancid, are highly inflammatory, and should be avoided.

Plant-based fats include avocado, avocado oil, coconut oil, extra-virgin olive oil, and MCT oil.

TEA FOR IMMUNITY

Rich in antioxidants and polyphenols, tea calms inflammation and boosts immunity. Chamomile soothes an anxious mind, rooibos provides allergy relief, and peppermint calms the belly. Oolong is particularly restorative, as it contains an amino acid called L-theanine, known to lower the risk of neurodegenerative diseases such as Alzheimer's and Parkinson's.

Teas include those made with astragalus, anise seed, ashwagandha, cat's claw, chaga mushroom, chai, chamomile, cinnamon, echinacea, elderberry, eucalyptus, ginger root, gingko, ginseng, hibiscus flower, horsetail mushroom, jasmine, lemongrass, licorice root, linden flower, mangosteen, matcha, moringa, olive leaf, oolong, pau d'arco, peppermint, raspberry leaf, reishi mushroom, rooibos, rosehip, rosemary, sage, spirulina, stinging nettle, tulsi, turmeric, valerian, white tea, and yerba mate.

Green tea is loaded with the antioxidant ECGC but can increase T-helper cells type 2, so I advise moderation and generally do not recommend it for individuals with severe allergies, allergic asthma, hay fever, acid reflux, Graves' disease, or eczema.

NATURAL SWEETENERS

Items in this category include apple butter, applesauce (unsweetened), brown rice syrup, coconut sugar, date sugar, local raw honey, maple syrup (100 percent pure), pumpkin purée, and stevia.

BAKING INGREDIENTS

Items in this category include almond extract, arrowroot flour, baking powder (without cornstarch), baking soda (without aluminum), carob powder, gelatin powder, cassava flour, coconut flour, tigernut flour, and vanilla extract.

MISCELLANEOUS

Items in this category include capers, *cocoa powder, coconut aminos, collagen peptides powder, coffee (in moderation), fish sauce, olives, *hummus, *paleo ketchup, *dark chocolate (at least 75 percent dark), dry red wine (limited to 5 ounces daily), unsweetened sparkling water, vegan pesto, vegan protein powder (soy-free), and vegetable and chicken broths (low sodium).

7-DAY SAMPLE MEAL PLAN

	DAY 1	DAY 2	DAY 3	DAY 4	DAY 5	DAY 6	DAY 7
Breakfast	Steel-cut oats (gluten-free) with pecans and blueberries	Kale, pineapple, and banana smoothie	Overnight chia seed breakfast bowl with berries	Gluten-free sourdough toast with almond butter served with seasonal fruit	Blueberry-avocado smoothie	Bone broth or miso soup with carrots, celery, and broccoli	Gluten-free toast with nut butter and a banana
Snack	Oolong tea, fresh pear, and almonds	Bone broth and a handful of almonds	Herbal tea and apple slices with almond butter	Herbal tea, berries, and walnuts	Bone broth and rice cake with avocado	Herbal tea, coconut yogurt with blueberries and raw honey	Herbal tea, strawberries, and almonds
Lunch	Turkey burger on a paleo bun with avocado and paleo ketchup	Wild salmon served with brown rice and black beans	Turkey breast, steamed broccoli, and half a sweet potato with olive oil dressing	Chopped salad with fennel and orange slices	Salad with lettuce, avocado, radishes, chicken, olive oil	Quinoa salad with chicken, grapes, and almonds	Chicken salad with arugula, avocado, sunflower seeds, broccoli sprouts, and olive oil
Snack	Kombucha tea, snap peas, and carrot sticks	Sliced cucumber and guacamole	Bone broth, rice cake with avocado	Celery sticks with hummus	Herbal tea and kale chips	Baby carrots and pumpkin seeds	Bone broth, rice cakes and guacamole
Dinner	Baked salmon and roasted brussels sprouts	Ground turkey served in romaine lettuce cups	Baked halibut and oven-roasted root veggies	Stir-fry shrimp*, carrots, broccoli, and bok choy	Baked chicken, brown rice, and spring mix salad	Shirataki yam noodles served with roasted cauliflower and onion	Wild salmon served with butternut squash "pasta" and vegan pesto

For autoimmune-friendly cookbooks and where to find specific ingredients mentioned in this chapter, please refer to the Resources section at the back of this book.

16

GUT-HEALING SUPPLEMENTS

*True health begins with your thoughts. Thinking about comfort, strength,
flexibility, and youthfulness attracts those qualities into your life and body.*

– Christiane Northrup, MD

A wealth of anti-autoimmune health benefits can be derived from just eating the right healthy foods. Adding the proper probiotics and supplements are especially therapeutic during the healing process, as they help repair the gut and manage inflammation. Following are some of the supplements I most often recommend to my patients. I encourage you to work with your functional medicine expert in selecting the proper supplements and dosages that are right for you.

Aloe vera (oral) is a succulent plant containing over 200 active components, including enzymes, antioxidants, fatty acids, folate, and choline, and vitamins A, C, and E. Likewise, it is one of the few plants that contain vitamin B12 and minerals like calcium, chromium, selenium, magnesium, manganese, potassium, sodium, and zinc. In the same family as onion and garlic, aloe supplements also contain acemannan, a polysaccharide that has been shown to be especially healing for those with constipation, IBS, rheumatoid arthritis, lupus, and type 1 diabetes. Recommended dosage is 50 mL daily. Be aware that higher dosages can be dangerous.

Coenzyme Q10 is a natural antioxidant and essential co-factor for the mitochondria of the body. It protects cells, plays an important role in metabolism, and helps your body clear reactive oxygen species, which would otherwise cause oxidative or inflammatory injury. While repairing, I recommend this because it helps restore T-cell balance and reduce inflammation. Dosage ranges from 50 mg to 1,200 mg.

Curcumin is another natural anti-inflammatory. As the main ingredient in turmeric, curcumin plays a critical role in cooling inflammation. Three types of curcumin have been clinically studied to be effective in decreasing inflammation—Theracurmin, Bcm-95, and Meriva—so I recommend one that contains one of these.

L-Glutamine is the most abundant amino acid in the body. However, glutamine stores are depleted during oxidative stress such as trauma, sepsis, and inflammatory bowel diseases. A number of recent studies have shown that taking it in supplement form helps suppress pro-inflammatory signaling pathways. Taken daily for thirty days, L-glutamine has shown to help heal leaky gut by sealing tight junctions. Among other things, it is especially helpful for managing irritable bowel syndrome, supporting thyroid function, and controlling sugar cravings. Be aware, however, that taking too much can bring on unwelcome symptoms such as gas, bloating, nausea, headache, dizziness, fatigue, itchiness, and more, so it's best to consult with your practitioner to determine the right dosage for you.

Glutathione is a powerful antioxidant and a critical regulator of oxidative stress and immune function. Found in every cell in the body, glutathione binds free radicals and toxins and ushers them out of the body. Our bodies naturally produce glutathione, but our stores can be depleted during times of oxidative stress such as trauma, poor diet, exposure to toxins, medications, and illness, thus triggering an inflammatory response. Studies show this supplement is particularly therapeutic for those with rheumatoid arthritis, Crohn's disease, and multiple sclerosis. I usually recommend three months of glutathione daily and one month off. Though most oral forms of glutathione are poorly absorbed, I have found that one version to be quite effective. Trizomal Glutathione by Apex Energetics contains NAC (the precursor to glutathione) and two forms of glutathione in a liposomal delivery. Starting dosage is 5 mL, once a day for adults, which can be increased to 5 mL twice a day.

Lipid Replacement Therapy is an oral supplement containing antioxidants and cell membrane phospholipids. This supplement mends damaged and oxidized mitochondria and restores cellular function, and is especially helpful for those living with chronic fatigue. Recommended dosage is usually between 1,000 to 3,000 mg. The brand I prefer is BodyBio PC, taken as two capsules once to twice a day.

Probiotics positively influence your immune function by targeting intestinal epithelial cells, mononuclear phagocytes, innate lymphoid cells, T and B cells, and regulatory T cells, which together perform a key role in immunity and maintaining oral tolerance. Probiotics work by introducing good bacteria that compete for nutrients with pathogens like *salmonella, Shigella,* or *E. coli.* In short, the good bugs starve out the bad.

Probiotics also stop bad bacteria from binding to the intestinal lining, increase the absorption of iron and B vitamins, decrease gut permeability to large molecules, and restore the microbiome after antibiotic use. Probiotic strains include *Saccharomyces boulardii, lactobacillus GG, L. plantarum, L. rhamnosus,* and *Bifidobacterium.* I typically start with a high dose of 100 billion CFUs of a bifido-lacto blend, and then taper down to 20 billion CFU as maintenance once the clinical goals are achieved.

MitoQ is another antioxidant that targets damaged mitochondria and delays disease progression. In mouse studies, it shows promise for alleviating pathogenesis in multiple sclerosis. My typical recommendation is two capsules daily.

Omega-3 fatty acids possess supreme anti-inflammatory effects and contain eicosapentaenoic acid (EPA) and docosahexaenoic acid (DHA). EPA aids in reducing cellular inflammation, neuroinflammation, triglycerides, and polysaturated fats. DHA comprises 90 percent of the brain's omega-3 fats and approximately half of the plasma in its neurons. It's worth noting that neuron loss accounts for numerous brain disorders.

Happily, DHA rejuvenates neurons and, consequently, lowers the risk of Alzheimer's disease. And finally, omega-3s help decrease LDL (so-called "bad cholesterol") while increasing HDL (beneficial cholesterol). In food sources, you'll find omega-3s in cold-water fish, walnuts, flaxseed, algae, and other good fats. Recommended dosage is 1,000 mg to 1,500 mg, two to three times a day.

Vitamin A is a fat-soluble nutrient, which means it's best absorbed when taken with a fatty food such as avocado. Stored in fatty tissues (particularly in the liver), vitamin A helps combat infection and treat eye issues and skin disorders like acne, eczema, and psoriasis. Metabolites such as retinoic acid (or retinol found in many skin care products to care for acne and bring evenness back to aging skin) in vitamin A is abundant in carrots, squash, leafy greens, liver, and eggs.

These are important elements in mucosal immune homeostasis, promoting the induction and expansion of T cells, particularly the ever-important T regulatory cells. Vitamin A also helps calm inflammation by preserving the cells that line the respiratory and digestive tract. I suggest vitamin A during the repair phase until the leaky gut can be stabilized, because it protects the cells in the gut lining. Recommended daily dosages will depend on your individual condition and need but will typically range between 5,000 and 20,000 IU a day. It's important to note that prolonged high-dose intake of supplemental vitamin A can lead to adverse effects and become toxic, so again, make sure you consult with your functional medicine expert first.

Vitamin B12 promotes immune balance, improves mood, protects your brain, and plays an essential role in red blood cell production and DNA synthesis. This essential nutrient also maintains the protective sheath around myelin nerves, which is particularly beneficial for those living with multiple sclerosis. When B12 is ingested, it is separated from food proteins by enzymes in the stomach. If there aren't enough enzymes (caused by breakdown of the hairlike villi in the small intestine), this process is hindered and the B12 will not travel to the small intestine for absorption. That means if your digestive tract is not intact, you may experience B12 deficiencies. Be sure to consult with your physician about the right form and dose of B12, as it varies significantly based on methylation genetics. I typically recommend 1,000 mcg daily.

Vitamin C protects cells and fights free radicals that lead to oxidative stress. Studies show that inadequate vitamin C intake can disrupt your immune function, including T cell and B cell function, and natural killer cytotoxic activity (which patrols for virus-infected cells). Vitamin C levels tend to be very high in leukocytes, but these deplete rapidly during infections. As a result, low levels of vitamin C can lead to cell death and immune suppression. One study opens the possibility of daily supplementation with 500 mg of vitamin C for the induction of oral tolerance to various food antigens, for example, gliadin, and of central tolerance against autoantigens.

Vitamin D3 and vitamin K2 (MK-7) work synergistically and should always be taken together to optimize the flow of calcium through the body. They should also be taken with high-fat foods, since vitamin D is fat-soluble. With the arrival of COVID-19, we heard a lot of news about the health benefits of vitamin D. But even before that, vitamin D received superstar status in the media, lauded for its restorative, supportive, and revitalizing role in immune functioning. Still, up to 75 percent of Americans remain deficient in vitamin D. This is mostly because we cannot obtain this crucial vitamin in food itself and it must be ingested via supplementation or from sunlight through the skin.

Vitamin D is not actually a vitamin but a hormone, and it helps protect against various autoimmune disorders, enhances the antimicrobial properties of monocytes and macrophages, and increases the body's defense against invading microorganisms. What's more, vitamin D can directly modify B cells into producing antibodies and reduce their differentiation into plasma cells and memory B cells, thus contributing to the inhibition of many autoimmune disorders. Since most of us are deficient in vitamin D, daily supplementation is recommended across the board.

When restoring tolerance, I recommend 2,000 to 50,000 IU, depending on the level of deficiency. Once your health is back in order, I recommend a daily dose of 2,000 to 4,000 IU. Since vitamin D is stored in fat tissues, it's easy to take too much, so ideally your levels should be monitored every three to six months by your functional medicine physician.

Vitamin E is another fat-soluble vitamin high in antioxidants. It is first absorbed in the intestines before traveling to the liver to be used or stored for future use. Because autoimmunity fractures the digestive system, this vitamin often cannot be absorbed properly, so replenishing its stock is important during your repair phase. Vitamin E protects lipid membrane and cells from free radicals. It also helps blood flow easily through blood vessels. It's best to get vitamin E from food, as long-term supplementation comes with its own set of health risks. Vitamin E is found abundantly in leafy greens, salmon, trout, avocado, nuts, and seeds.

AFTERWORD

Science and medicine continually evolve. What we understand about disease today clearly dwarfs what we knew just twenty years ago. Such progress requires us to see things in new or different ways, and this is how we can most effectively tackle problems. In medicine, this is true in the world of autoimmune and inflammatory disorders. Sadly, these conditions still reside in the gray zone of traditional Western medicine. Only a very small minority of medical schools include anything about the topics discussed in this book in their curriculum, but this will rapidly change because we plainly have no other choice.

When I graduated from medical school in 2008, our main nutritional education included which diet to select for our patients while they were in the hospital. How can diet, something that has such a profound effect on our health and well-being, be so overlooked in the medical community? The good news is, this is changing. Because it has to.

As I write this, the world is beginning its transition out of the COVID-19 pandemic. But even before this dreaded virus, we were a world overwhelmed with epidemic proportions of autoimmune disease—not just in people middle-aged and older but in young adults and children as well. Throw COVID-19 into the mix, and we are now seeing even more people with autoimmune issues. Known as long-haulers, these people continue to experience symptoms months after recovering from a COVID-19 infection, most notably a development of autoimmunity against their lungs. At the time of this writing, one study estimates that up to 10 percent of those who have had COVID experience long-term symptoms. Other published studies indicate that upwards of 80 percent of patients continue to have troublesome symptoms like brain fog and fatigue three months after the onset of COVID-19—many weeks and months after testing negative for the virus.

Think about that: Long after the COVID-19 infection itself has cleared, autoimmunity against the body persists. If we sit back and wait to see how our immune systems will respond to these ever-growing threats, we will lose this battle. We have to take matters into our own hands and fight back. If our food is inadvertently attacking us, we change what we eat. If the chemicals in our environment are killing us and the other animals that we share this planet with, then we have to find another way. If viruses become more deadly and transmittable in an effort to co-inhabit this world with us, then we need to understand how to protect ourselves more than ever before.

Cancer, heart attacks, stroke, dementia, diabetes, and autoimmune disease are the leading causes of adult death on this planet. Leaky gut has been linked in the scientific literature to all of these diseases. When we address our gut health, we begin to heal.

If I can impart just one important truth to you after reading this book, it's that your health is in your hands. Your body is not a runaway train. On the contrary: By being conscious of what you put in your body and understanding the individual needs of your unique immune system, you ultimately have the power to direct that train wherever you want. It all boils down to treating yourself with care. By following the steps outlined in this book, you can execute the most crucial and effective means of taking control of your health and steering it in the direction YOU choose.

Cheers and in good health,
Elroy Vojdani, MD, IFMCP
Los Angeles, California
May 2021

ACKNOWLEDGMENTS

Countless people were instrumental in the creation of this book. First and foremost, my father Aristo Vojdani, PhD, who taught me and many other doctors everything we know about the immune system. Thank you for your endless dedication and passion in helping me and the world be better versions of what we are.

My wife, Tiffany Vojdani, an incredibly strong and beautiful soul. When I came home from the hospital frustrated and defeated by the way medicine works these days, you always pushed me to find another way. I would never be where I am without you.

A special thank you to my mother, Georgette Vojdani, PsyD. From day one, you told me to be unapologetically me and taught me how to survive difficult days.

And to my beautiful daughters, Jade and Raya. Every day is sunshine with you.

And finally, I want to thank my patients. I am so proud of each and every one of you. This book exists for you and others like you.

GLOSSARY

Archaea are microorganisms that are similar to bacteria in size and simplicity of structure but differ in lipid composition.

Adaptive immunity, also called specific or acquired immunity, produces an immune response to a very specific pathogen. The adaptive immune response is meant to attack non-self pathogens but can sometimes make errors and attack itself.

Agglutinin is an antibody, lectin, or other substance that causes particles such as bacteria, blood cells, and antigens to coagulate and aggregate.

Allergy is a damaging immune response that targets otherwise non-threatening foreign substances such as pollen, pet dander, or a particular food such as milk, eggs, peanuts, tree nuts, fish, crustacean shellfish, wheat, and soy.

Amino acids are a group of small, nitrogen-containing molecules that combine to form proteins. In the human body, there are twenty amino acids total: nine are essential and eleven are nonessential.

Antibiotics are drugs designed to prevent, inhibit, or destroy microorganisms such as bacteria, yeast, and fungi. They can lead to a breakdown in gut integrity, as they also kill beneficial microorganisms.

Antibodies are defensive Y-shaped blood proteins produced by white blood cells in response to the presence of a specific non-self antigen. They are designed to recognize and attach to foreign substances in the body, including bacteria and viruses. *See also* autoantibodies and immunoglobulins.

Antigen is a molecule or molecular structure present on the outside of a pathogen that produces an immune response in the body, namely the production of antibodies.

Aquaporin is a mechanism within a cell that allows water to enter and exit in a continuous flow.

Autoantibody is an antibody that reacts against a person's own body, or "self" tissues.

Autoimmunity occurs when the immune system goes awry and attacks the body's own tissues.

B cells, also called B lymphocytes, are a type of white blood cell produced in the bone marrow.

Bacteria are single-celled organisms with a tough protective coating called an antigen, which is designed to resist white blood cells. Though much smaller than a human or plant cell, bacteria can have a mighty effect on the body, both good and bad.

Basophils are a type of white blood cell.

Beta-casomorphin-7 (BCM-7) is a milk peptide with opioid characteristics and has been detected in the urine and blood samples of patients with neurological disorders. BCM-7 peptides can cause changes in the digestive tract, immune function, and brain development as well.

Biologics are synthetic antibodies that bind to cytokines and remove them from the bloodstream. Unfortunately, patients who take biologics lose an arm of their immune system and become prone to infection and are at higher risk for developing leukemia, lymphoma, and melanoma.

Blood-brain barrier (BBB) is a protective sheath around the brain that controls which substances are allowed in and out of the brain.

Body burden of chemicals refers to an accumulation of synthetic chemicals that have built up in body tissues over a period of time.

Carbamylated proteins (anti-CarP) are peptides associated with rheumatoid arthritis.

Capillaries are branching blood vessels that form networks throughout the body and drain into the veins. They are so small that a single blood cell can barely pass through them. They are responsible for exchanging nutrients, gases, and waste products between body tissue and blood.

Casein is a milk protein.

Central tolerance is a mechanism in the thymus that trains the cells of the immune system to recognize "self" tissue from "non-self." It begins to develop in babyhood and takes about two or three years to fully develop.

Circulatory system circulates blood, oxygen, hormones, and nutrients throughout the body and helps remove waste products. It features the heart, arteries, blood vessels, and capillaries. It also includes the lymphatic system, which circulates lymph fluid throughout the body.

Claudins (from the Latin claudere "to close") are proteins found in the tight junctions. Some claudins help to "tighten" tight junctions, while others selectively allow paracellular transport of certain ion species, or "loosen" tight junctions as needed.

Citrullination occurs when the amino acid arginine is converted to another non-essential amino acid called citrulline. For people with rheumatoid arthritis, this process alters type-2 collagen.

Cross-reactivity. *See* molecular mimicry.

Cytokines are glycoproteins secreted by various cells in the body, mainly cells of the immune system, including T-helper cells.

Cytolethal distending toxins (CDTs) are bacterial toxins that damage DNA in targeted cells.

DNA, or deoxyribonucleic acid, is a self-replicating molecule that carries an individual's genetic information. It consists of two polynucleotide chains that coil around each other to form a double helix.

Dendritic cells act as messengers to other cells. They become increasingly important once the adaptive immune system develops.

Dysbiosis results when bad bacteria in the gut outweigh the good.

Enzymes are molecules (most of which are proteins) that bind to other molecules and alter them in some way. They act as biological catalysts to create a particular chemical reaction in the body.

Endotoxins, the byproducts of infection, are toxins located inside a bacterial cell. When the cell disintegrates, the toxin is released. *See also* exotoxins.

Eosinophils are inflammatory white blood cells that target larger pathogens like parasitic worms. They're also responsible for allergic responses.

Epitope is the site on an antigen to which an antibody attaches. *See also* paratope.

Epithelial layer is a single layer of protective cells that lines the gastrointestinal tract and separates the gut from the bloodstream.

Exotoxins are toxins secreted by bacteria outside the cell. *See also* endotoxins.

Food immune reactivity is an immunoglobulin G (IgG) or immunoglobulin A (IgA) response controlled by T and B cells. Classic examples include celiac disease (CD) and non-celiac gluten sensitivity (NCGS). Unlike food allergies, which are immediate, food immune reactions usually occur four to seventy-two hours after exposure.

Gliadin is an insoluble protein present in gluten. There are four types of gliadin, classified by their amino sequence as alpha, beta, gamma, and omega (α, β, γ, and ω). Some research has found that gliadin affects the human brain. *See also* gluten *and* glutenin.

Glomerular basement membrane is a protein in the filtration system of the kidneys, with the resulting autoimmune response causing glomerulonephritis, an acute inflammatory response in the kidney.

Glucosaminoglycans are a group of compounds located in connective tissue. They play a role in cell signaling and help regulate cell growth, anticoagulation, and wound repair. *See also* proteoglycans.

Gluten is a binding protein in cereal grains, especially wheat. It comprises two proteins—gliadin and glutenin. *See also* gliadin *and* glutenin.

Glutenin is a soluble protein present in gluten. The adhesive properties in glutenin are responsible for the elastic texture in baked goods such as bread. *See also* gluten *and* gliadin.

Granulocyte-macrophage colony-stimulating factor (GM-CSF) is a cytokine secreted by macrophages, T cells, mast cells, natural killer cells, endothelial cells, and fibroblasts. Studies show the GM-CSF plays a role in regulating intestinal and inflammatory responses.

Gut barrier. *See* intestinal barrier.

Gut-brain axis describes the relationship between the gut and the brain. Recent studies have shown the that microbes in the gut microbiota influence these interactions.

Gut-skin axis describes the relationship between the gut and the skin. Research has linked gut health to skin homeostasis.

T-helper cells release inflammatory cytokines and stimulate B cells to make more antibodies. They differentiate into specific subtypes, including Th1, Th2, Th3, Th9, Th17, or TFH, all of which facilitate distinct types cytokines and immune responses.

Homeostasis is a state in which all body systems are stable and in balance.

Human herpesvirus 6 (HHV-6) is a member of the herpesvirus family. There are over 130 species of herpesvirus, of which there are eight known to infect humans. Between 25 to 95 percent of most populations are infected with HHV-6 by the age of three, and most individuals are asymptomatic. HHV-6 reactivation is most common in individuals with a compromised immune system. Though more research is needed, some researchers speculate that HHV-6 is linked to chronic fatigue syndrome. Latent HHV-6 and HHV-7 are both more prevalent in the blood of fibromyalgia patients.

Human leukocyte antigen (HLA) is a key molecule found on the surface of most cells in the body. It plays an important role in the immune system response to foreign invaders.

Increased intestinal permeability. *See* leaky gut syndrome.

Immune cells are a collection defensive cells in the immune system that fight against invading pathogens. They develop from stem cells in the bone marrow and go on to become different of white blood cells.

Immune response occurs when the immune system is activated.

Immune system comprises the biological structures and processes within an organism that protects against disease. To function properly, an immune system must detect a wide variety of agents, from viruses to parasitic worms and distinguish them from the organism's own healthy tissue. Disorders of the immune system can result in autoimmune disease, inflammatory disease, and cancer.

Immunoglobulins, also known as IG, are Y-shaped globular blood proteins produced by white blood cells (WBCs) after initial exposure to a specific disease antigen. They identify and neutralize foreign substances such as pathogenic bacteria, viruses, and toxins. *See* antibodies.

Indole-3-carbinol is a healing chemical compound that helps regulate mucosal immune function. It is found in abundance in cruciferous vegetables, leaves, and sprouts.

Innate immunity is sometimes called non-specific immunity because it attacks anything it perceives as an intruding pathogen. Present at the time of birth, it is the body's first line of defense and relies on inflammatory cytokines released by T-helper cell types 1 (Th1), 17 (Th17), and others.

Intestinal barrier, also known as the gut barrier, is the mucosal wall of the gut. It acts as a barrier between the contents of the gut and the bloodstream and is lined by epithelial cells, tight junctions, capillaries, and intestinal flora.

Intestinal permeability describes the control of material passing from inside the gastrointestinal tract through the cells lining the gut wall. Tight junctions in the gut wall act like microscopic doors that selectively open to allow water and nutrients into the bloodstream and close to block anything harmful. When this process is increased, the integrity of the gut is lost, allowing larger molecules to enter the bloodstream. *See also* leaky gut syndrome.

Intestinal wall, through which nutrients pass.

Junctional adhesion molecules (JAMs) are glycoproteins that regulate tight junction formation.

Leaky gut syndrome is a term used to describe increased intestinal permeability. It results when the epithelial layer of the gut lining is damaged and tight junctions are compromised by inflammation. Gaps in the damaged gut lining allow macromolecules—food proteins, bacteria, yeast, and other toxic compounds—into the bloodstream where they don't belong. When this happens, the immune system perceives a foreign invader and launches an attack.

Lectins, proteins that are part of a plant's natural defense system, appear in high concentrations in cereal grains, beans, seeds, nuts and potatoes. Adverse effects on humans may include nutritional deficiencies, immune or allergic reactions, gastrointestinal distress, and leaky gut. Many lectins can be disabled by soaking, sprouting, and fermenting.

Leukocytes, also known as white blood cells, are part of the immune system's defense against infectious disease and foreign materials.

Lewy bodies are abnormal aggregations of protein that develop inside nerve cells affected by Parkinson's disease.

Lipopolysaccharides (LPS) are large-molecule endotoxins that increase gut permeability and allow the passage of lectins, food antigens, and bacterial toxins into the circulation. Once in the circulatory system, if they are not removed within two to four minutes by Kupffer cells, LPS can induce potent pathophysiological effects in humans. Elevated LPS component levels in the blood have been associated with conditions such as Alzheimer's, multiple sclerosis, inflammatory bowel disease, diabetes, cardiovascular disease, Parkinson's, autism, depression, and many autoimmune disorders.

Lymphatic system makes up a vital part of the immune system and consists of thin tubes (known as lymph vessels) and oval-shaped tissues called lymph nodes.

Lymphocytes are white blood cells in the adaptive immune system. They include natural killer (NK) cells, T cells, and B cells.

Lysozyme is an enzyme that damages bacterial cell walls.

Macrophages are a subtype of a phagocyte, also known as a "eating cells." Together with neutrophils, they are collectively the Pac-Man of the immune system, gobbling up harmful organisms and infected cells as they circulate through the bloodstream.

Mast cells are a class of white blood cells that release histamine and live in the mucosal lining of the sinuses, throat, lungs, and digestive system.

Microbiome is a community of bacteria, fungi, and viruses that populate a particular environment. In the human body, 70 percent of the microbiome resides in the gut, where it plays a key role in the immune system.

Microorganism, also known as a microbe, is a microscopic organism that may consist of a single cell or more than one cell.

Molecular mimicry occurs when a food protein contains a sequence of amino acids similar to the structure of a person's own tissue. The result is often the development of food immune reactivity.

Mucous membrane is a protective epithelial tissue that secretes mucus and lines several body cavities and internal organs, including the eyelids, mouth, nose, trachea, lungs, and digestive tract. Its role is to protect the body from potentially harmful outside substances.

Myelin is a fatty substance that forms a layer over some nerve axons. It allows the nerves to transmit signals, and, when damaged, gradually produces weakness associated with loss of reflexes.

Myelin basic protein (MBP) is a foundational protein of the nervous system, contributing to the outer-layer protection (referred to as a sheath) of nerve cells.

Myelin oligodendrocyte glycoprotein (MOG) is a glycoprotein in the central nervous system.

Natural killer (NK) cells are a type of white blood cell that targets tumors, cancer cells, and body cells infected with pathogens.

Neuroautoimmunity is an immune inflammatory disease of the nervous system.

Neurodegeneration is a degeneration of the nervous system, particularly the neurons in the brain.

Neuroinflammation is an inflammatory response within the nervous system. It can be the result of an infection, toxicity, or traumatic brain injury.

Neutrophils are a subtype of a phagocyte. Like macrophages, they circulated through the bloodstream engulfing invading pathogens.

Nightshade plants belong to the *Solanaceae* plant family. Nightshade fruits, vegetables, and spices include white potatoes, tomatoes, tomatillos, eggplant, bell peppers, goji berries, cayenne pepper, chili peppers, paprika, curry, and chili powder. Due to their high levels of lectin, they can be problematic for some people living with autoimmunity.

NSAIDs: Nonsteroidal anti-inflammatory drugs are a class of drugs that provide fever reduction and anti-inflammatory effects. Frequent and long-term use of NSAIDs contributes to increased intestinal permeability.

Occludin is an enzyme protein and one of the main component proteins of tight junctions.

Oral tolerance is a subtype of peripheral tolerance responsible in suppressing the immune response against harmless antigens in food. Established in the womb at the earliest stage of human development, oral tolerance is the result of your immune system learning to recognize necessary and nonpathogenic substances that enter through the oral route for metabolization.

Oxidative stress is an imbalance between free radicals and antioxidants. Over time, an overabundance of free radicals damages fatty tissue, DNA, and proteins in the body.

Paratope is an antigen-binding site located on each arm of the Y-shaped antibody. This is what allows the antibody to bind to the epitopes of an invading antigen. As a visual aid, think of the paratope as a lock and the epitope as a specific key. *See also* epitope.

Peptides is a short chain of amino acids connected by peptide bonds. Peptides are the building blocks of proteins such as collagen, elastin, and keratin.

Peripheral tolerance is a branch of central tolerance. Peripheral tolerance ensures that self-reactive T cells that escape into the periphery are deleted or become anergic (functionally unresponsive to antigen).

Phagocytes also known as "eating cells." Phagocytes include two subtypes—macrophages and neutrophils. Think of them collectively as the Pac-Man of the immune system, gobbling up harmful organisms and infected cells as they circulate through the body.

Phosphorylated tau is a protein in the brain that plays a key role in the development of neuroautoimmunity.

Probiotics are live bacteria and yeasts that are beneficial for the digestive system.

Proteoglycans are macromolecules present in connective tissue that bonds to glycosaminoglycans.

Proteus mirabilis is a species of bacteria found in the urinary tract. When immunoglobulin M (IgM) antibodies against it show up in a blood test, in suggests a pathogenic relationship to rheumatoid arthritis.

Regulatory T cells (Tregs) act as the immune system's police force, patrolling the circulatory system, supporting immune homeostasis, and inducing tolerance between friendly bacteria and food antigens.

Short-chain fatty acids (SCFAs) provide energy to colon cells, help regulate inflammation, and buttress the intestinal wall against invading pathogens.

Stem cells have the ability to give rise to more cells—either more stem cells or a wide variety of specialized cells. They live in the bone marrow and form white blood cells, including T and B cells.

T cells are a type of white blood cell and play a vital role in the adaptive immune system. They begin life in the bone marrow but migrate to the thymus to mature. In the thymus, T cells are put through rigorous training that force them to recognize "self" antigens from "non-self" antigens. Those that fail this testing are destroyed in the thymus. Those that pass leave the thymus to enter the circulatory system.

T3 (triiodothyronine) is a powerful hormone made in the thyroid gland. It contains three iodine molecules in its structure and affects nearly every process in the body, including body temperature, metabolism, and heart rate. *See* T4 (thyroxine) *and* thyroid hormone (TH).

T4 (thyroxine) is the main hormone produced by the thyroid gland. It contains four iodine molecules in its structure. Along with T3, it affects the entire body. In the liver and certain tissues of the brain, some T4 lose an atom and are converted into T3. *See* T3 (triiodothyronine) *and* thyroid hormone (TH).

Tight junctions, also known as zonulae occludentes, are composed of the proteins zonulin, occludin, claudin, and junctional adhesion molecules (JAM). They are closely associated areas of two adjacent cells whose membranes join together to form a virtually impenetrable barrier. Tight junctions act like portals to the body while the intestinal epithelial lining prevents unwanted trespassers from entering the bloodstream. Think of them as microscopic doors that selectively open to allow water and nutrients into the bloodstream and close to block anything harmful.

Thyroid hormone (TH) refers to T3 and T4 collectively.

Thyroid peroxidase (TPO) is an essential enzyme in the thyroid responsible for making T4 and T3.

Thyroid-stimulating hormone (TSH) is a messenger chemical produced in the pituitary gland. TSH only binds to receptors on cells in the thyroid. The amount of TSH the pituitary makes depends on how much T4 is circulating throughout the bloodstream. If it is very little, the pituitary will produce more TSH. This is how it tells the thyroid to produce more T4. Once T4 reaches a comfortable level, the pituitary gland shuts off its production of TSH.

Thyroid-stimulating immunoglobulins (TSI) are an autoantibodies that can bind to receptors in the thyroid gland, resulting in Graves' disease over time.

TSH receptor antibodies (TSHRab), also known as thyroid-stimulating immunoglobulins, cause autoimmune hyperthyroidism, namely Graves' disease.

Thymus is a small gland located above the heart. Composed of lymphoid tissue, the thymus is large in newborn babies and shrinks in size as we age. The thymus plays a key role in the maturation of T cells.

Thyroid peroxidase (TPO) is an enzyme that plays a critical role in the production of T4 and T3.

Transglutaminase is an enzyme that forms strong bonds between glutamine and lysine proteins and plays a role in blood clotting. It is ubiquitous in various tissues throughout the body. In blood tests, autoantibodies against transglutaminase 2 (tTG2) show up for gut issues, transglutaminase 6 (tTG6) presents for brain, and for skin, it's tTG3. Transglutaminase derived from yeast, fungi, and plants, as well as from the plasma of pigs and cows is used as a food and meat glue in food processing.

Vagus nerve links the brain to the digestive system and runs from the brain to the face and thorax to the abdomen.

Villi are small, hairlike projections in the epithelial layer that facilitate the passage of fluids and nutrients in the intestines.

White blood cells (WBC), also called leukocytes, are the cells of the immune system. These include T and B cells, monocytes, neutrophils, basophils, and eosinophils.

Yersiniosis is an infection caused by undercooked pork.

NOTES

Zonulin is a protein that modulates the permeability of tight junctions.

REFERENCES

The following is provided for those who would like to check a fact or dig deeper into the topics covered in this book. Most of the peer-reviewed academic articles are available online. Simply go to www.doi.org and enter the digital object identifier (DOI) or run a Google search of the article title.

Abbott A (2016). "Scientists bust myth that our bodies have more bacteria than human cells." Nature. DOI: 10.1038/nature.2016.19136

Aburto N J, Ziolkovska A, Hooper L, Elliott P, Cappuccio F P, Meerpohl J J et al (2013). "Effect of lower sodium intake on health: systematic review and meta-analyses." *British Medical Journal*. DOI: 10.1136/bmj.f1326

American Thyroid Association, The (ATA). "General Information." www.thyroid.org/media-main/press-room/

Bengmark S (2007). "Advanced Glycation and Lipoxidation End Products—Amplifiers of Inflammation: The Role of Food." *Journal of Parenteral and Enteral Nutrition.* DOI: 10.1177/0148607107031005430

Bercik P, Verdu EF, Foster JA, Macri J et al (2010). "Chronic gastrointestinal inflammation induces anxiety-like behavior and alters central nervous system biochemistry in mice." *Gastroenterology*. DOI: 10.1053/j.gastro.2010.06.063

Bloomfield SF, Rook GAW, Scott EA, Shanahan F et al (2016). "Time to abandon the hygiene hypothesis: new perspectives on allergic disease, the human microbiome, infectious disease prevention and the role of targeted hygiene." *Perspectives in Public Health*. DOI: 10.1177/1757913916650225

Boyd DB (2003). "Insulin and Cancer." *Integrative Cancer Therapies*. DOI:10.1177/1534735403259152

Braak H, Rub U, Gai WP (2003). "Idiopathic Parkinson's disease: possible routes by which vulnerable neuronal types may be subject to neuroinvasion by an unknown pathogen." *Journal of Neural Transmission*. DOI: 10.1007/s00702-002-0808-2

Bredesen, DE (2017). *The End of Alzheimer's: The First Program to Prevent and Reverse Cognitive Decline*. Avery Publishing.

Brigham & Woman's Hospital (2003). "Facts About RA." Brigham and Woman's Hospital Rheumatoid Arthritis Sequential Study. brassstudy.org

Briney B, Inderbitzin A, Joyce C et al (2019). "Commonality despite exceptional diversity in the baseline human antibody repertoire." *Nature*. DOI: 10.1038/s41586-019-0879-y

Brookmeyer, R (2017). "Forecasting the prevalence of preclinical and clinical Alzheimer's disease in the United States." *Alzheimer's & Dementia: The Journal of the Alzheimer's Association*. DOI: 10.1016/j.jalz.2017.10.009

Bucala R, Mitchell R, Arnold K et al (1995). "Identification of the major site of apolipoprotein B modification by advanced glycosylation end products blocking uptake by the low density lipoprotein receptor." *Journal of Biological Chemistry*. DOI: 10.1074/jbc.270.18.10828

Cecil DL, Johnson K, Rediske J et al (2005). "Inflammation-induced chondrocyte hypertrophy is drive by receptor for advanced glycation end products." *The Journal of Immunology*. DOI:10.4049/jimmunol.175.12.8296

Centers for Disease Control and Prevention (2011-2012). "National Survey of Children's Health." The National Electronic Health Records Survey. www.cdc.gov/nchs/slaits/nsch.htm

Chanda ML, Levitin DJ (2013). "The neurochemistry of music." *Trends in Cognitive Science*. DOI: 10.1016/j.tics.2013.02.007

Charlton S, Ramsøe A, Collins M et al (2019). "New insights into Neolithic milk consumption through proteomic analysis of dental calculus." *Archaeological and Anthropological Sciences*. DOI: 10.1007/s12520-019-00911-7

Coppen JJW (1995). "Non-wood forest products 6: Gums, resins and latexes of plant origin." Food and Agriculture Organization of the United Nations. http://www.fao.org/3/v9236e/v9236e.pdf

Davis C (2013). "From passive overeating to 'food addiction': a spectrum of compulsion and severity." *ISRN Obesity*. DOI: 10.1155/2013/435027

Eby GA, Eby KL (2010). "Magnesium for treatment-resistant depression: a review and hypothesis." *Medical Hypotheses*. DOI: 10.1016/j.mehy.2009.10.051

Faraco G, Brea D, Garcia-Bonilla L, Wang G et al (2018). "Dietary salt promotes neurovascular and cognitive dysfunction through a gut-initiated TH17 response." *Nature Neuroscience*. DOI: 10.1038/s41593-017-0059-z

Forsyth CB, Shannon KM, Kordower JH et al (2011). "Increased intestinal permeability correlates with sigmoid mucosa alpha-synuclein staining and endotoxin exposure markers in early Parkinson's disease." *Plos One*. DOI: 10.1371/journal.pone.0028032

Frank M (2015-2021). "ADHD: The Facts." Attention Deficit Disorder Association. https://add.org/adhd-facts/

Gerbault P, Liebert A, Itan Y, Powell A et al (2021). "Evolution of lactase persistence: an example of human niche construction." *Philosophical Transactions of the Royal Society*. DOI: 10.1098/rstb.2010.0268

Ghoshal UC, Shukla R, Ghoshal U (2017). "Small Intestinal Bacterial Overgrowth and Irritable Bowel Syndrome: A Bridge between Functional Organic Dichotomy. *Gut and Liver*. DOI: 10.5009/gnl16126

Hawkes CH, del Tredici K, Braak H (2007) "Parkinson's disease: a dual-hit hypothesis." *Neuropathology and Applied Neurobiology*. DOI: 10.1111/j.1365-2990.2007.00874.x

Heuser G, Vojdani A (2008). "Enhancement of natural killer cell activity and T and B cell function by buffered vitamin C in patients exposed to toxic chemicals: the role of protein kinase-C." *Immunopharmacology and Immunotoxicology.* DOI:10.3109/08923979709046977

Hodsdon W, and Zwickey H (2010). "Reproducibility and Reliability of Two Food Allergy Testing Methods." *Natural Medicine Journal.* naturalmedicinejournal.com

Jankiewicz A, Aulepp H, Altmann F et al (1998). "Serological investigation of 30 celery-allergic patients with particular consideration of the thermal stability of IgE-binding celery allergens." *Allergo Journal International,* vol 7:87-95.

Kim MH, Kim H (2017). "The Roles of Glutamine in the Intestine and Its Implication in Intestinal Diseases." *International Journal of Molecular Sciences.* DOI: 10.3390/ijms18051051

Kleinewietfeld M, Manzel A, Titze J et al (2013). "Sodium chloride drives autoimmune disease by the induction of pathogenic Th17 cells." *Nature.* DOI: 10.1038/nature11868

Koppel BS, Harden CL, Daras M (1991). "Tegretol excipient-induced allergy." *Archives of Neurology.* DOI: 10.1001/archneur.1991.00530200025008

Lambert J, Mejia S, Vojdani A (2019). "Plant and human aquaporins: pathogenesis from gut to brain." *Immunologic Research.* DOI: 10.1007/s12026-018-9046-z

Lauretti E, Nenov M, Dincer O, Iuliano L, Praticò D (2019). "Extra virgin olive oil improves synaptic activity, short-term plasticity, memory, and neuropathology in a tauopathy model." *Aging Cell.* DOI: 10.1111/acel.13076

Leckie RL, Oberlin LE et al (2014). "BDNF mediates improvements in executive function following a 1-year exercise intervention." *Frontiers in Human Neuroscience.* DOI: 10.3389/fnhum.2014.00985

Lerner A, Matthias T (2015). "Food Industrial Microbial Transglutaminase in Celiac Disease: Treat or Trick." *International Journal of Celiac Disease.* DOI: 10.3389/fnhum.2014.00985

Lerner A, Matthias T (2015). "Changes in intestinal tight junction permeability associated with industrial food additives explain the rising incidence of autoimmune disease." *Autoimmunity Reviews.* DOI: 10.1016/j.autrev.2015.01.009.

Lerner A, Jeremias P, Matthias T (2015). "The World Incidence and Prevalence of Autoimmune Diseases Is Increasing." *International Journal of Celiac Disease.* DOI: 10.12691/ijcd-3-4-8

Lowry MD, Hudson CF, Callen JP (1994). "Leukocytoclastic vasculitis caused by drug additives." *Journal of the American Academy of Dermatology.* DOI: 10.1016/S0190-9622(94)70097-4

Lull C, Wichers HJ, Savelkoul HF (2005). "Antiinflammatory and immunomodulating properties of fungal metabolites." *Mediators of Inflammation.* DOI: 10.1155/MI.2005.63

Lyte M, Varcoe JJ, Bailey MT (1998). "Anxiogenic effect of subclinical bacterial infection in mice in the absence of overt immune activation." *Physiology & Behavior*. DOI: 10.1016/S0031-3384(98)00145-0

Ma WT, Chang C, Gershwin ME, Lian ZX (2017). "Development of autoantibodies precedes clinical manifestations of autoimmune diseases: A comprehensive review." *Journal of Autoimmunity*. DOI: 10.1016/j.jaut.2017.07.003

Maes M, Kubera M, Leunis JC (2008). "The gut-brain barrier in major depression: intestinal mucosal dysfunction with an increased translocation of LPS from gram negative bacteria (leaky gut) plays a role in the inflammatory pathophysiology of depression." *Neuro Endocrinology Letters*.

Mari A (2002). "IgE to cross-reactive carbohydrate determinants: analysis of the distribution and appraisal of the in vivo and in vitro reactivity." *International Archives of Allergy and Immunology*. DOI: 10.1159/000067591

McCann D, Barrett A, Copper A, Crumpler D et al (2007). "Food additives and hyperactive behavior in 3-year-old and 8/9-year-old children in the community: a randomized, double-blinded, placebo-controlled trial." *The Lancet*. DOI: 10.1016/S0140-6736(07)61306-3

Mikkelsen H, Larsen JC, Tarding F (1978). "Hypersensitivity reactions to food colours with special reference to the natural colour annatto extract (butter colour)." *Archives of Toxicology*, vol. 1. DOI: 10.1007/978-3-642-66896-8_16

Haghighat N, Rajabi S, Mohammadshahi M (2021). "Effect of synbiotic and probiotic supplementation on serum brain-derived neurotrophic factor level, depression and anxiety symptoms in hemodialysis patients: a randomized, double-blinded, clinical trial." *Nutritional Neuroscience*. DOI: 10.1080/1028415X.2019.1646975

Neutra MR, Kraehenbuhl J-P (2005) "Chapter 7: Cellular and molecular basis for antigen transport across epithelial barriers." *Mucosal Immunology*, vol. 1, eds. Mestecky, Lamm, Strober, Bienenstock, McGhee, Myer. DOI: 10.1016/B978-012491543-5/50011-5

Parodi A, Paolino S, Greco A, Drago F et al (2008). "Small intestinal bacterial overgrowth in rosacea: clinical effectiveness of its eradication." *Clinical Gastroenterology and Hepatology*. DOI: 10.1016/j.cgh.2008.02.054

Phillips RJ, Walter GC, Wilder SL et al (2008). "Alpha-synuclein-immunopositive myenteric neurons and vagal preganglionic terminals: autonomic pathway implicated in Parkinson's disease?" *Neuroscience*. DOI: 10.1016/j.neuroscience.2008.02.074

Polito CA, Cai ZY, Shi YL et al (2018). "Association of Tea Consumption with Risk of Alzheimer's Disease and Anti-Beta-Amyloid Effects of Tea." *Nutrients*. DOI: 10.3390/nu10050655

Rajaei E, Mowla K, Ghorbani A, Bahadoram S et al (2016). "The effect of omega-3 fatty acids in patients with active rheumatoid arthritis receiving DMARDs therapy: double-blind randomized controlled trial." *Global Journal of Health Science*. DOI: 10.5539/gjhs.v8n7p18

Richter J, Benson V, Grobarova V, Svoboda J et al (2010). "CD161 receptor participates in both impairing NK cell cytotoxicity and the response to glycans and vimentin in patients with rheumatoid arthritis." *Clinical Immunology.* DOI: 10.1016/j.clim.2010.03.005.

Rodriguez, Tori (2013). "Gut Bacteria May Exacerbate Depression." *Scientific American Mind.* www.scientificamerican.com/article/gut-bacteria-may-exacerbate-depress/

Rolph GM (2012). *Something About Sugar; Its History, Growth, Manufacture and Distribution.* Hardpress Publishing.

Rook GAW, Martinelli R, Brunet LR (2003). "Innate immune responses to mycobacteria and the downregulation of atopic responses." *Current Opinion in Allergy and Clinical Immunology.* DOI: 10.1097/00130832-200310000-00003

Rosenkranz MA, Davidson RJ et al (2013). "A comparison of mindfulness-based stress reduction and an active control in modulation of neurogenic inflammation." *Brain, Behavior, and Immunity.* DOI: 10.1016/j.bbi.2012.10.013.

Saçma M, Geiger H (2021). "Exercise generates immune cells in bone." *Nature.* DOI: 10.1038/d41586-021-00419-y

Sander I, Raulf-Heimsoth M, Weimer K et al (2006). "Sensitization due to Gum Arabic (Acacia senegal): The Cause of Occupational Allergic Asthma or Crossreaction to Carbohydrates?" *International Archives of Allergy and Immunology.* DOI: 10.1159/000094182

Savidge TC, Sofroniew MV, Neunlist M (2007). "Starring roles for astroglia in barrier pathologies of gut and brain." *Laboratory Investigation.* DOI: 10.1038/labinvest.3700600

Scudellari M (2017). "Cleaning up the hygiene hypothesis." *Proceedings of the National Academy of Sciences of the Unites States of America* (PNAS). DOI: 10.1073/pnas.1700688114

Senior BW, McBride PD, Morley KD, Kerr MA (1995). The detection of raised levels of IgM to Proteus mirabilis in sera from patients with rheumatoid arthritis. *Journal of Medical Microbiology.* DOI: 10.1099/00222615-43-3-176

"Sodium and Food Sources" (2013). Centers for Disease Control and Prevention (CDC). www.cdc.gov/salt/food.htm

Strazzullo P, D'Elia L, Kandala N-B, Cappuccio FP (2009). "Salt intake, stroke, and cardiovascular disease: meta-analysis of prospective studies." *British Medical Journal.* DOI: 10.1136/bmj.b4567

Tobacman JK (2001). "Review of harmful gastrointestinal effects of carrageenan in animal experiments." *Environmental Health Perspectives.* DOI: 10.1289/ehp.01109983

Tsao TM, Tsai MJ, Hwang JS et al (2018). "Health effects of a forest environment on natural killer cells in humans: an observational pilot study." *Oncotarget.* DOI:10.18632/oncotarget.24741

Universität Bayreuth (2021). "Biologists investigate effects of bisphenols on nerve cells." *ScienceDaily*. www.sciencedaily.com

University of California, San Diego Health Sciences (2012). "Potential new drug therapy for Crohn's disease." *ScienceDaily*. www.sciencedaily.com

Uribarri J, Woodruff S, Goodman S et al (2010). "Advanced Glycation End Products in Foods and a Practical Guide to Their Reduction in the Diet." *Journal of the American Dietetic Association*. DOI: 10.1016/j.jada.2010.03.018

U.S. Department of Health and Human Services (2005). "Progress in Autoimmune Disease Research." *National Institutes of Health*. www.niaid.nih.gov/sites/default/files/adccfinal.pdf

Van Bever HP. Docx M, Stevens WJ (1989). "Food and food additives in severe atopic dermatitis." *Allergy: European Journal of Allergy and Clinical Immunology*. DOI: 10.1111/j.1398-9995.1989.tb04205.x

Vernon PJ, Loux TJ, Schapuro NE et al (2013). "The Receptor for Advanced Glycation End Products Promotes Pancreatic Carcinogenesis and Accumulation of Myeloid-Derived Suppressor Cells." *The Journal of Immunology*. DOI: 10.4049/jimmunol.1201151

Vernon LL, Dillon J, Steiner ARW (2009). "Proactive coping, gratitude, and posttraumatic stress disorder in college women." *Anxiety, Stress, & Coping: An International Journal*. DOI: 10.1080/10615800802203751

Visser S, Holbrook J, Danielson M et al (2014). "Epidemiology of attention-deficit/hyperactivity disorder: national and state-based patterns and opportunities for policy evaluation." Paper presented at the ADHD Summit, Baton Rouge, LA.

Vojdani A (2009). "Detection of IgE, IgG, IgA and IgM antibodies against raw and processed food antigens." *Nutrition & Metabolism*. DOI: 10.1186/1743-7075-6-22

—, Lambert J (2011). "The Role of Th17 in Neuroimmune Disorders: Target for CAM Therapy. Part II." *Evidence-Based Complementary and Alternative Medicine*. DOI: 10.1093/ecam/nep063

—, Turnpaugh C, Vojdani E (2018). "Immune reactivity against a variety of mammalian milks and plant-based milk substitutes." *Journal of Dairy Research*. DOI: 10.1017/S0022029918000523

—, Vojdani C (2015). "Immune reactivities against gums." *Alternative Therapies in Health and Medicine*. 21 (Supplement 1): 64-72

—, Kharrazian /d, Mukherjee PS (2014). "The Prevalence of Antibodies against Wheat and Milk Proteins in Blood Donors and Their Contribution to Neuroimmune Reactivities." *Nutrients*. DOI: 10.3390/nu6010015

—, Turnpaugh CC (2020). "Antibodies against Group A Streptococcus, dopamine receptors, and ganglioside GM1 cross-react with a variety of food antigens, potentially interfering with biomarkers for PANS and PANDAS." *Biomarkers in Neuropsychiatry*. DOI: 10.1016/j.bionps.2020.100023

—, Afar D, Vojdani E (2020). "Reaction of Lectin-Specific Antibody with Human Tissue: Possible Contributions to Autoimmunity." Journal of Immunology Research. DOI: 10.1155/2020/1438957

NOTES

NOTES

RESOURCES

ADDITIONAL READING

Detox Your Home, Christine Dimmick

Gluten Freedom, Alessio Fasano, MD

Grain Brain, David Perlmutter, MD, and Kristin Loberg

Missing Microbes, Martin J. Blaser, MD

The Easy Autoimmune Protocol Cookbook, Karissa Long and Katie Austin

The End of Alzheimer's, Dale E. Bredesen, MD

The Gut Health Guidebook, Sarah Ballantyne, PhD

The Healing Kitchen, Alaena Haber, MS, OTR, and Sarah Ballantyne, PhD

The Plant Paradox, Steven R. Gundry, MD

INGREDIENT SOURCES

Local Harvest will help you find your local farmers market. *localharvest.org*

ShopAIP is an online grocery store specializing in autoimmune protocol foods and is a fantastic place to start for those with allergies, food sensitivities, and proinflammatory diseases. *shopaip.com*

Oregon Valley Farm is a small family business dedicated to sustainable, ethically raised, and humanely slaughtered beef, pork, and chicken products that are antibiotic- and hormone-free. They also offer subscription boxes for delivery. *oregonvalleyfarm.com*

Thrive Market is a grocery delivery service that operates on a subscription membership. They offer wholesale food, including staples, grass-fed beef, pasture-raised pork, organic chicken, and wild-caught seafood. *thrivemarket.com*

Wild Alaskan Company is a great resource if you lack a good fishmonger in your community. The company operates on a monthly membership plan and offers a wide variety of flash-frozen, wild-caught, and sustainable species from Alaska and the Pacific Northwest, including sockeye salmon, Coho salmon, Pacific cod, Pacific halibut, and wild Alaska pollock. *wildalaskancompany.com*

Bone Broth

Bonafide Provisions offers a selection of slow-simmered, collagen-rich bone broths with no preservatives. They use nothing but purified water, organic garlic and onions, Celtic salt, and bones from grass-fed, pasture-raised animals (and some chicken feet). *bonafideprovisions.com*

Kettle & Fire combines humanely raised, 100 percent grass-fed marrow bones with premium organic vegetables and filtered water. It contains no additives, preservatives, antibiotics, hormones, artificial flavors, artificial colors, or sodium. *kettleandfire.com*

Dairy Alternatives

Almond Cow is for those who prefer to control the ingredients that go into their alternative milks by making their own. Starting at $215, the machine is an investment; however, the benefits are huge, as you avoid plastic packaging and the gums, sweeteners, and other objectionable ingredients typically found in store-bought alternative milks. The company also offers a recipe book to make soups, infusions, dressings, vegan butter, ice cream, pulpmeal dishes, and more. *almondcow.co*

Forager Project is an organic, certified vegan, non-dairy milk alternative made with cashews and no added soy, gluten, sugar, food gums, or oils. Visit their website to find a store near you that carries the product. *foragerproject.com*

MALK carries a line of sprouted, vegan-friendly milk alternatives made from almonds, cashew, and oats. Bottled in BPA-free containers, the various non-dairy milks contain no soy, GMOs, or food gums. To find a store that carries this product, visit *malkorganics.com*

Miyoko's European-Style Cultured Vegan Butter melts, spreads, browns, and bakes like real butter—but more important, it tastes like it, too. Cultured and churned in California's Sonoma County, this vegan product is made with coconut oil, cashew milk, sunflower oil, organic sunflower lecithin, and sea salt. It is free of lactose, palm oil, gluten, soy, and GMO products. *miyokos.com*

Gluten-Free Bread and Pasta

Jovial Foods boasts a selection of organic, gluten-free pastas. In addition to being gluten-free, their products contain no nuts, legumes, gums, or starch. The company offers free shipping on orders over $99. *jovialfoods.com*

Young Kobras offers a selection of gluten-free sourdough breads made with unrefined flours, and is also egg-, gum-, and dairy-free. Ingredients are mostly organic and consist of water, brown rice flour, sorghum flour, millet flour, cassava flour, psyllium husk, and sea salt. Tastes best toasted. The company is located in San Francisco but ships nationwide. *youngkobras.com*

SUPPLEMENT BRANDS

BodyBio PC is a lipid replacement therapy containing non-GMO, pure liposomal phospholipid complex. *bodybio.com*

EnteroVite delivers short-chain fatty acids (SCFAs) that support intestinal mucosal health and microbiota diversity. *apexenergetics.com*

MegaSporeBiotic is a spore-based, broad-spectrum probiotic shown to maintain healthy intestinal barrier function. This formula promotes microbial diversity. *microbiomelabs.com*

RepairVite includes flavonoids, carotenoids, and phytochemicals that are known to nourish gastrointestinal tissue. It includes extracts with mucilage content and uses glycoproteins that help sustain the mucous membrane. *apexenergetics.com*

Trizomal Glutathione features a liposomal solution to deliver S-acetyl L-glutathione (SAG), combined with reduced glutathione (GSH), and N-acetyl L-cysteine (NAC). This formulation utilizes three ways to support glutathione—intracellular with SAG, intracellular biosynthesis with NAC, and extra/intracellular (systemic) support with GSH. *apexenergetics.com*

TESTING LABORATORIES

Cyrex Laboratories
2602 South 24th Street
Phoenix, AZ 85034
(877) 772-9739
cyrexlabs.com

Doctor's Data
3755 Illinois Avenue
St. Charles, IL 60174-2420
(800) 323-2784
doctorsdata.com

Great Plains Laboratory
11813 West 77th Street
Lenexa, KS 66214
(800) 288-0383
greatplainslaboratory.com

Labcorp
531 South Spring Street
Burlington, NC 27215
(800) 833-3984
abcorp.com

Quest Diagnostics
500 Plaza Drive
Secaucus, NJ 07094
(866) 697-8378
questdiagnostics.com

StrateGene
3140 Mercer Avenue
Bellingham, WA 98225
(800) 547-9812
strategene.me

BIOGRAPHY

Dr. Elroy Vojdani is a pioneer in the field of functional medicine and the founder of Regenera Medical, a boutique functional medicine practice in Los Angeles, California. Warmly referred to as "Dr. V" by his patients, he is a licensed medical doctor and an Institute for Functional Medicine Certified Practitioner (IFMCP). Taking an innovative approach, Dr. Vojdani combines his medical training and knowledge with scientifically proven methods and state-of-the-art lab testing to accurately diagnose and treat chronic medical conditions.

A native of Southern California, Dr. Vojdani grew up in Los Angeles. At the tender age of three, he eagerly spent time in the laboratory with his father and role model, Aristo Vojdani, PhD—who is regarded as "the father of functional immunology." Dr. V fondly recalls receiving the gift of a microscope from his father, which he then regularly used during summer school breaks spent in the lab running experiments with his father. Before entering first grade, Dr. V helped his father prepare for national and international lectures on immunology, health, and science. Though these lectures were for educators and practitioners, Dr. V often quietly sat in the back of the conference hall to listen to his father's presentations.

During high school, Dr. V was a star athlete on the football team. After fracturing his ankle, he landed in the hospital—an experience that ignited his dream of becoming a doctor. Upon graduating from medical school at the University of Southern California and completing his residency at USC's Keck School of Medicine, Dr. V began his career as an interventional radiologist—diagnosing and surgically treating complex, late-stage cancers and other extremely debilitating diseases. While this experience gave him unique insights into how radiology testing is conducted and interpreted, his desire to prevent or effectively treat disease—by finding and addressing the root cause—remained his core purpose for practicing medicine.

Today, he continues in his father's footsteps—pioneering to find answers for chronic medical conditions that are often misdiagnosed or undiagnosed and/or mistreated/untreated. Each day, Dr. V meets patients who are at their wits' end from trying to find the cause of their chronic medical conditions. Drawing upon his medical training, his background in radiology, and his deep understanding of how blood tests are created and conducted, Dr. Vojdani utilizes his extensive knowledge and experience to accurately diagnose patient conditions, and then create a customized and effective treatment plan. His goal is to accurately identify and heal chronic medical conditions before they irreversibly consume the patient's life.

Highly respected by his peers, Dr. V is well published in medical journals, and he lectures regularly at medical science–related symposiums. His groundbreaking published research on the causes of Alzheimer's is changing the way the medical community regards this debilitating disease. Today, more than 44 million people worldwide currently suffer from dementia—a number that is projected to triple in the next 30 years. The results of Dr. V's new research, combined with a simple blood test that he helped create, are helping people in their 40s and 50s find out if they are at risk of developing the disease, and how they can take measures to slow down the progress—or avoid it altogether.

Dr. V is passionate about sharing his functional medicine teachings and practices with the world and believes that this life-changing form of medicine should be the future of health care.

When he isn't helping patients, Dr. V enjoys traveling, hiking, spinning, yoga, cooking, and spending time with his wife and two daughters. He's also an avid reader of medical science journals to stay up-to-date on the latest advancements and news.

For additional information, please visit www.regeneramedical.com.

INDEX

biologics, 62, 63
bisphenol A (BPA), 94
bisphenol S (BPS), 95
Blaser, Martin J., 28, 29
blood cells, 15, 21, 22, 35, 38, 51, 62, 82
blood-brain barrier (BBB), 30, 38, 47, 52, 53
body burden of chemicals, 17
bone broth, 41, 48, 74, 101, 105
bowel movement, 42, 48
brain fog, 2, 7, 19, 28, 29, 37, 38, 41, 46, 48, 50,
52, 65, 77-79, 101
Bredesen, Dale E., 123
Brigham RA Sequential Study (BRASS), 61
bromelain, 48

C

C-section, 46, 70
campylobacter jejuni, 44, 45, 52
carbamylated proteins (anti-CarP), 116
carob gum. *See also* food gums, 93
carrageenan. *See also* food gums, 93, 102
cartilage, 61, 62, 64
casein, 18, 34, 50, 82, 94, 101
Centers for Disease Control and Prevention
(CDC), 49
celiac disease, 15, 18, 20, 34, 35, 43, 44, 46, 61,
68, 69, 79, 80, 82, 94, 101
central tolerance, 23, 109
cereal grains. *See* grains, 46, 77, 88
chemical, 15-17, 20, 21, 29, 35, 45, 48, 51, 55,
63, 74, 77, 78, 90, 92
synthetic, 16, 17, 20, 34, 51, 58, 63, 75, 77, 92, 94
chlamydia, 65
claudins, 116
chronic inflammatory demyelinating
polyneuropathy (CIDP), 21, 51
citrullinated peptides. *See* citrullination, 63, 64
citrullination, 62, 64
coconut, 40, 41, 83, 91, 102-105
aminos, 104
flour, 102, 104
milk, 41, 102
sugar, 40, 91, 104
coenzyme Q10, 107
collagen, 48, 62, 63, 82, 101, 104
corn, 17, 36, 37, 39, 40, 45, 46, 51, 52, 56-58, 70,

78, 79, 85, 87-89, 92, 94, 100, 103
corticosteroids, 65
COVID-19, 3, 58, 109, 111
Crohn's disease, 20, 43, 44, 67, 80, 82, 84
cross reactivity. *See also* molecular mimicry, 46, 50,
52, 79, 93
cruciferous vegetables, 45, 99, 100
curcumin, 56, 107
Cyrex Laboratories, 2, 36-38, 46, 52, 58, 64, 70
Array 2 Intestinal Antigenic Permeability Screen,
36, 52, 58, 70
Array 3X Wheat/Gluten Proteome Reactivity
and Autoimmunity, 36, 52, 58, 70
Array 4 Gluten-Associated Cross-Reactive Foods
and Foods Sensitivity, 36, 46, 52, 58
Array 5 Multiple Autoimmune Reactivity Screen,
36
Array 7 Neurological Autoimmune Reactivity,
37, 52
Array 8 Joint Autoimmune Reactivity Screen,
37, 64
Array 20 Blood Brain Barrier Permeability Screen,
37, 52
ELISA, 35, 37
GAM total serum immunoglobulins. *See also*
laboratory testing, 38
cytokines, 21-24, 36, 50, 62, 63, 67
cytolethal distending toxins (CDTs), 44

D

dairy. *See also* milk. 2-4, 11, 18, 33, 36-41, 45-48, 51,
52, 56, 58, 62, 64, 68-70, 73, 81-85, 93, 94, 102
alternatives, 102, 132
and autoimmunity, 82
DDT, 77, 94
dendritic cells, 22
depression, 7, 9, 15, 28, 29, 42, 46-53, 58, 65, 75,
78, 87, 88, 99
dermatitis herpetiformis (DH), 20, 68, 69
dermatomyositis, 20
diabetes. *See also* type 1 diabetes. 2, 3, 15, 17, 70,
75, 90, 111
discoid lupus erythematosus (DLE), 20, 69
disease-modifying antirheumatic drugs
(DMARDs), 63
DNA, 42, 3, 16, 22, 92, 100, 109

Made in the USA
Las Vegas, NV
26 May 2022